SETON HALL UNIVERSITY

3 3073 10360876 4

Handbook of

Polytrauma Care

and Rehabilitation

D1714420

SETON HALL UNIVERSITY
UNIVERSITY LIBRARIES
SOUTH ORANGE, NJ 07079

Handbook of Polytrauma Care and Rehabilitation

David X. Cifu, MD
Chairman and Herman J. Flax, M.D. Professor
Department of Physical Medicine and Rehabilitation
Executive Director, Center for Rehabilitation Sciences and
  Engineering
Virginia Commonwealth University
Richmond, Virginia

National Director for Physical Medicine and Rehabilitation
  Services
U.S. Department of Veterans Affairs
Washington, DC

Henry L. Lew, MD, PhD
Professor, John A. Burns School of Medicine
University of Hawaii at Manoa
Honolulu, Hawaii

Rehabilitation Consultant
Defense and Veterans Brain Injury Center (DVBIC)
Professor, Department of Physical Medicine and Rehabilitation
Virginia Commonwealth University
Richmond, Virginia

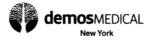
demosMEDICAL
New York

RC
552
P67
C54
2014

Visit our website at www.demosmedpub.com

ISBN: 9781936287550
e-book ISBN: 9781617051005

Acquisitions Editor: Beth Barry
Compositor: diacriTech

© 2014 Demos Medical Publishing, LLC. All rights reserved. This book is protected by copyright. No part of it may be reproduced, stored in a retrieval system, or transmitted in any form or by any means, electronic, mechanical, photocopying, recording, or otherwise, without the prior written permission of the publisher.

Medicine is an ever-changing science. Research and clinical experience are continually expanding our knowledge, in particular our understanding of proper treatment and drug therapy. The authors, editors, and publisher have made every effort to ensure that all information in this book is in accordance with the state of knowledge at the time of production of the book. Nevertheless, the authors, editors, and publisher are not responsible for errors or omissions or for any consequences from application of the information in this book and make no warranty, expressed or implied, with respect to the contents of the publication. Every reader should examine carefully the package inserts accompanying each drug and should carefully check whether the dosage schedules mentioned therein or the contraindications stated by the manufacturer differ from the statements made in this book. Such examination is particularly important with drugs that are either rarely used or have been newly released on the market.

Library of Congress Cataloging-in-Publication Data
Cifu, David X.
  Handbook of polytrauma care and rehabilitation / David X. Cifu, Henry Lew.
    p. ; cm
  Includes index.
  ISBN 978-1-936287-55-0 — ISBN 978-1-61705-100-5 (ebook)
1. Post-traumatic stress disorder—Patients—Rehabilitation.
2. Psychic trauma—Patients—Care. 3. Traumatic neuroses—Patients—Rehabilitation.
I. Lew, Henry L., author. II. Title.
  RC552.P67C54 2014
  616.85'21–dc23
                    2013020955

Special discounts on bulk quantities of Demos Medical Publishing books are available to corporations, professional associations, pharmaceutical companies, health care organizations, and other qualifying groups. For details, please contact:

Special Sales Department
Demos Medical Publishing, LLC
11 West 42nd Street, 15th Floor
New York, NY 10036
Phone: 800-532-8663 or 212-683-0072
Fax: 212-941-7842
E-mail: specialsales@demosmedpub.com

Printed in the United States of America by Gasch Printing.
13 14 15 16 17 / 5 4 3 2 1

Contents

Preface

With advancements in body armor technology and battle-field trauma care, the health care system is faced with an increasing number of combat survivors who have sustained a combination of multiple physical injuries and psychological trauma. In a 2005 directive, the Veterans Health Administration (VHA) coined the term polytrauma to describe *"injury to the brain in addition to other body parts or systems resulting in physical, cognitive, psychological, or psychosocial impairments and functional disability"* (Department of Veterans Affairs, Veterans Health Administration Directive, 2005) (1).

There are many textbooks on critical care and traumatic brain injury (TBI), as well as physical medicine and rehabilitation (PM&R), which health professionals have relied on to take care of this growing cohort of military service members and veterans with polytrauma. In the context of clinical care and effective teaching, the authors felt the need to develop a practical, pocket-sized handbook that focuses on polytrauma care and rehabilitation. This handbook was written in a reader-friendly style, with succinct text and flow charts to highlight the key concepts.

While the extent of recovery from TBI often guides the overall rehabilitation process, other comorbidities are equally important. The individual chapters focus on common conditions that polytrauma patients present with, including medical/physical issues (aphasia, burns, contractures, dysphagia, focal weakness, headache, hearing dysfunction, neglect, neuroendocrine dysfunction, neurogenic bowel/bladder, postconcussive syndrome, posttraumatic seizure, pressure ulcers, sexual dysfunction, spasticity, visual dysfunction) and psychological issues, such as depression, posttraumatic stress disorder (PTSD). Vocational issues (ability to return to work) are also discussed. The goals are to (1) summarize the most frequent problems encountered by these patients and (2) offer a roadmap for clinicians regarding how to initiate and navigate through the continuum of care in order to achieve the best possible outcome.

The Defense and Veterans Brain Injury Center (DVBIC) has been working collaboratively with the Department of Veterans Affairs (VA) and the Department of Defense (DOD) to provide continuing education for health professionals in the care of patients with polytrauma. The authors would like to thank the DVBIC leadership and staff for their continued dedication to improve the diagnosis and treatment of our wounded warriors.

REFERENCE

1. Department of Veterans Affairs, Veterans Health Administration Directive. Polytrauma Rehabilitation Centers. Washington (DC): Veterans Health Administration; 2005, June 8, p. 2.

Polytrauma Basics

1

What Is
Polytrauma?

1. Conservative estimates of the incidence for traumatic brain injury (TBI) range from 1.5 to 3.0 million annually, with 80%–95% being mild in severity (ie, a concussion). While most of these injuries will have progressive recovery in the months to years after injury with excellent long-term functional outcomes, the impact of a TBI alone is usually sufficient to significantly challenge the injured individual, their family and the clinicians providing their care. Even injuries that are initially mild in severity can present with marked physical, cognitive, and behavioral dysfunction that requires considerable time and clinical expertise to recover. When a significant secondary injury (eg, amputation, burn, spinal cord injury, fracture) or medical/psychological disorder (eg, posttraumatic stress disorder, depression, generalized anxiety disorder, substance use) occurs, the

resulting "polytrauma" can have profound effects that greatly compound that seen with a TBI alone. Similarly, individuals who incur repeated TBIs (even mild TBIs) within a relatively short period of time (eg, less than 1 year apart) can have both short- and long-term difficulties that are significantly worse than would have been expected.

2. In military conflict, polytrauma is far more common than civilian injury, although the multiple injuries of polytrauma are seen in both settings. The recent conflicts in Afghanistan and Iraq generated TBIs in nearly 10% of all combat-deployed service members and polytrauma was seen in more than 90% of these individuals with TBI. Fortunately, a rapid recognition of this injury type and the extent of functional deficits that could accompany such a complex injury allowed for the development of a comprehensive polytrauma care system in the military and Veteran Affairs health care system.

3. The hallmark of care for polytrauma (as with all but the least severe TBIs) is a patient-centered, interdisciplinary approach that works with the injured individual and the family to address all aspects of the injury as they impact the person's life. While the acute assessment and management of most traumatic injuries are well circumscribed and coordinated in both the military and civilian trauma systems, the initial period of recovery ("rehabilitation") that focuses on symptom management and a return to home independence is less standardized and consistently managed. Even less attention is paid to the long-term recovery of community reintegration, a return to productivity (work, school, leisure), and a focus on overall wellness.

4. While optimal care for polytrauma is delivered by compassionate, experienced, interdisciplinary teams of specialty clinicians with a holistic approach and an emphasis on patient engagement, the key to success lies in a thorough understanding of the types of difficulties seen and the effective means of managing them. Unfortunately, the research evidence supporting much of polytrauma rehabilitation is limited, thus consensus and expert opinion remain the state of the art for care.

2

Taking a History

1. Taking the history of a patient with polytrauma, including traumatic brain injury (TBI), can be challenging due to the complexity of the injury, assessments, symptoms, and treatments received, which may be challenging to fully recollect for the patient (especially in light of persistent cognitive limitations) and equally difficult to collect for the busy clinician. An organized approach is crucial, making sure to utilize as many data sources as are available, including family members.

2. The first area to be covered is **Injury Characteristics**, which includes
   - Etiology
     - Ground-level fall
     - Elevated-level fall
     - Low-speed motor vehicle collision (<25 MPH)
     - High-speed motor vehicle collision (>25 MPH)
     - Blunt trauma
     - Sports-related
     - Military-related (blast)
     - Penetrating injury

- Severity
  - Alteration or loss of consciousness
  - Posttraumatic amnesia
  - Computerized tomography (CT) scan findings (acute/chronic)
  - MRI scan findings (acute/chronic)
  - Glasgow coma score (lowest/best in first 24 hours)
  - Intracranial pressure readings
  - Abnormal brainstem reflex findings

3. The second area to be reviewed is **Past Medical History**, which includes;
   - Prior TBI
   - H/o psychiatric illness
   - H/o substance/alcohol abuse
   - H/o neurologic disorder
   - General medical survey
   - H/o surgery

4. The third area to be covered is a **Review of Symptoms**, which includes
   - Headaches—frequency, severity, duration, and if they most resemble migraine, tension type, or cluster headaches
   - Dizziness or vertigo—frequency
   - Weakness or paralysis—location, severity
   - Sleep disturbance—type and frequency, nightmares (associated with posttraumatic stress disorder [PTSD])
   - Fatigue—severity
   - Mobility—describe limitations
   - Balance—describe symptoms and limitations
   - Cognitive impairment—severity
     - Memory impairment
     - Slowness of thought
     - Confusion
     - Decreased attention

- – Difficulty concentrating
- – Difficulty understanding directions
- – Difficulty using written language or comprehending written words
- – Delayed reaction time
- Speech difficulties—severity and specific type of problem
  - – Aphasia—type, symptoms
  - – Dysarthria—type
- Swallowing difficulties—type, severity
- Pain—frequency, severity, duration, location, mediating factors
- Bowel problems—report type and frequency of need for assistance
- Bladder problems—report the type of impairment and the measures needed for maintenance
- Behavioral symptoms (include severity)
  - – Anxiety
  - – Depression/ mood swings
  - – Agitation
  - – Irritability
  - – Restlessness
  - – Disinhibition
  - – Hypervigilance (associated with PTSD)
  - – Paranoid thoughts (associated with PTSD)
- Sexual dysfunction—type
- Sensory changes—location and type
- Visual problems—describe
- Hearing problems—describe
- Decreased smell and/or taste
- Seizures—type and frequency
- Hypersensitivity to sound or light—describe
- Oral and dental problems—describe

5. The fourth area to be reviewed is **Medications**, which should include
- Prescription
  - Current
    - All
    - Psychotherapeutics
  - Former
    - Used for TBI-related issues
- Over the counter
  - Current, all
  - Former
  - Used for TBI-related issues
- Nutraceuticals/supplements
  - Current, all
  - Former
  - Used for TBI-related issues
- Allergies

6. The fifth area to be covered is **Social History**, which should include
- Education
  - Highest completed level
  - Learning disabilities
- Productivity
  - Current occupation
  - Prior occupation(s)
  - Military service
  - Disability
  - Hobbies
- Social supports
  - Married/significant other
  - Family

- Sexuality
  - Activity
  - Birth control
  - Orientation
7. The sixth area to be reviewed is **Functional History**, which should include
  - Mobility
    - Basic (bed, chair, balance)
    - Ambulation (assistive device, distance, safety)
    - Community (public transportation, private vehicle)
  - Activities of daily living
    - Basic (grooming, bathing, toileting, dressing)
    - Instrumental (cooking, laundry, homemaking, financial management)
  - Continence
    - Bladder
    - Bowel
  - Communication
    - Oral
      - Receptive
      - Expressive
    - Written
      - Literate

3

Performing a Physical Examination

OVERVIEW

1. Examining a patient with polytrauma, including a traumatic brain injury (TBI), can be challenging due to the complexity of the injury and assessments, symptoms, and treatments received, which may be challenging to fully recollect for the patient (especially in light of persistent cognitive limitations) and for the patient to fully tolerate. An organized approach is crucial and it may be both necessary and beneficial to stage the evaluation over the course of the day or even several days to ensure completeness.

2. The first area to be covered is **Cognition**, which includes:
   - Orientation
   - Command following (single, multistep)
   - Attention
   - Concentration
   - Memory (short and long term)

- Naming/repetition
- Abstract thinking
- Judgment

3. The second area to be covered is **Behavior**, which includes:
   - Depression
   - Anxiety
   - Irritability
   - Agitation
     - Restlessness
     - Disinhibition
     - Emotional lability

4. The third area to be covered is **Musculoskeletal**, which includes:
   - Manual muscle testing
   - Joint range of motion (including the temporomandibular joint)
   - General bone survey (to assess for occult fractures)
   - Muscle tone
   - Mobility
     - Balance (sitting, standing, dynamic)
     - Transfers
     - Gait (indoor, outdoor, stair)

5. The fourth area to be covered is **Neurologic**, which includes:
   - Cranial nerve testing
   - Sensory function
   - Special sensory
     - Vision
     - Hearing
     - Smell/taste
   - Muscle stretch reflexes
   - Brainstem reflexes

- Primitive reflexes (frontal release signs)
- Cerebellar testing
- Fine and gross motor coordination
  - Tremor
- Autonomic nervous system

6. The fifth area to be covered is a **General Medical** Exam, which includes:
   - Skin
     - Extremities (edema, erythema, pulses, cords)
     - Pressure points (occiput, elbow, trochanters, sacrum, buttocks)
   - Heart
   - Lung
   - Abdomen
   - Endocrine (thyroid)

DETAILED PROCEDURES IN PERFORMING A PHYSICAL EXAMINATION

Cognitive

1. **Orientation:** Ask the patient to name the place, date, and a specific person such as someone in the room, or the current president).

2. **Command following:** Single command (eg, raise your right hand), or multistep command (eg, put your left hand on your face and stick out your tongue).

3. **Attention and concentration:** These are assessed by the serial 7s test (asking the patient to subtract 100 by 7s. This can also be assessed by asking the patient to spell a five-letter word (such as WORLD) backward.

4. **Memory (short and long term):** The examiner can start by asking the patient to remember three objects; for

example, red ball, wrist watch, and blue car. Then the examiner can proceed with the rest of the interview and physical exam. Short-term memory is assessed by asking the patient to recall these three objects at the end of the visit. Long-term memory can be assessed by asking the patient to recollect well-known historical events in the patient's life, such as names of schools attended.

5. **Naming/repetition:** The patient's basic language ability can be assessed by asking him/her to name common objects, repeat words and phrases, as well by observing his/her spontaneous speech utterance.

6. **Abstract thinking:** This ability to decipher properties shared by specific items to conceptualize generalizations can be tested either visually or verbally. Verbal tests often involve inquiries on proverbs, such as "What does 'Don't cry over spilled milk' mean?" or "How are oranges and apples alike?" Patients who think concretely won't be able to explain beyond the obvious.

7. **Judgment:** The patient's ability to make appropriate decisions can be assessed by asking hypothetical but ecologically valid questions such as "If you found a letter addressed to someone else in your mail box, what would you do?"

Behavioral

1. **Depression:** Symptoms of depression include: insomnia, or excessive sleeping, suicidal thoughts or attempts, decreased energy, feelings of worthlessness, helplessness, hopelessness, pessimism, difficulty concentrating, irritability, restlessness, anhedonia, anorexia or hyporexia, and persistent sad, anxious, or "empty" feelings.

2. **Anxiety:** Symptoms of anxiety include feeling wound-up, tense, sleepless, irritable, or restless. The patient feels that his/her heart races, breathing increases, and muscles tense without any evident life-threatening event.

3. **Irritability:** The patient is noticed to often lose his/her temper, "having a short fuse," restless, and easily annoyed by others over trivial events. It is often associated with overtalkativeness, flight of ideas, and increased motor activity.

4. **Agitation:** Clinically, excessive aggression or agitation without bodily discomfort, influence important to rule out the underlying cause of agitation before initiating medical treatment.

5. **Restlessness:** There are basically two kinds of restlessness. Psychomotor restlessness refers to an excess of motor activity that is clearly manifested externally, while akathisia refers to unpleasant sensations of inner restlessness that manifest with an inability to sit still or remain motionless. The latter may be due to medication side effects, Parkinson's disease, or withdrawal from benzodiazepines.

6. **Disinhibition:** The inability to inhibit or control oneself may be manifested either behaviorally or emotionally. The impulsivity and poor risk assessment may resemble hypomania, showing aggressive outbursts and expression of uninhibited basic instincts such as hyperphagia and hypersexuality.

Musculoskeletal

1. **Manual muscle (strength) testing:** This is useful in determining the degree of muscle weakness from injury or disuse atrophy.

Manual Muscle Testing Grading System (0–5)

0	❏ None	No visible or palpable contraction
1	❏ Trace	Visible or palpable contraction with no motion (a1)
2	❏ Poor	Full ROM gravity eliminated
3	❏ Fair	Full ROM against gravity
4	❏ Good	Full ROM against gravity, moderate resistance
5	❏ Normal	Full ROM against gravity, maximal resistance

Abbreviation: ROM, range of motion.

2. **Joint range of motion (ROM):** The joint ROM refers to the degree to which a joint can move, as measured with a goniometer. Each joint has a normal ROM that can be found in online textbooks or publications. The normal ranges also vary with age.

3. **Muscle tone:** Patients with polytrauma may have either abnormally high muscle tone (hypertonia) or abnormally low muscle tone (hypotonia), depending on the location of injury. Hypertonia is seen in upper motor neuron diseases, presenting clinically as either spasticity or rigidity. Spasticity is velocity-dependent resistance to passive stretch, while rigidity is velocity-independent resistance to passive stretch. In clasp-knife response, there is increased resistance only at the beginning or at the end of the movement. Hypotonia is a manifestation of lower motor neuron disease. In flaccidity, the extremity appears floppy, and stretch reflex responses are decreased.

The Modified Ashworth Scale (below) is commonly used for grading spasticity.

Spasticity Grade	Clinical Manifestation of the Affected Part
0	No increase in muscle tone
1	Slight increase in muscle tone, manifested by a catch and release, or by minimal resistance at the end of the ROM during flexion or extension
1+	Slight increase in muscle tone, manifested by a catch, followed by minimal resistance throughout the remainder of the movement (less than 50%)
2	More marked increase in muscle tone through most of movement, but the affected part can be easily moved
3	Considerable increase in muscle tone, passive movement difficult to perform
4	Affected part is rigid in both flexion and extension

4. **Mobility, transfer, and locomotion:** A patient's mobility can be measured in the following categories:
   a. Transfers: Bed/chair/wheelchair
   b. Transfers: Toilet
   c. Transfers: Bathtub/shower
   d. Transfers: Car
   e. Locomotion: Walking/wheelchair

f. Locomotion: Stairs

g. Community mobility

The Functional Independence Measure (FIM™) scale assesses physical disability. This scale focuses on the burden of care—that is, the level of disability indicating the burden of caring for the afftected person. The FIM score ranges from 1 to 7, with 1 (total assistance) being the lowest possible score and 7 (complete independence) being the best possible score.

FIM Scoring Criteria

Score	Description
7	Complete independence, no helper is needed
6	Modified independence (patient requires use of a device, but no physical assistance), no helper is needed
5	Helper needed for supervision or setup
4	Helper needed for minimal contact assistance (patient can perform 75% or more of task)
3	Helper needed for moderate assistance (patient can perform 50%–74% of task)
2	Helper needed for maximal assistance (patient can perform 25%–49% of tasks)
1	Helper needed for total assistance (patient can perform < 25% of the task or requires more than 1 person to assist)

5. **Balance—static and dynamic:** Both static and dynamic balance can be obtained while the patient is standing and

sitting. The functional balance grades are categorized as follows:

Normal	**Static:** Patient able to maintain steady balance without handhold support
	Dynamic: Patient accepts *maximal challenge* and can shift weight easily within full range in all directions
Good	**Static:** Patient able to maintain balance without handhold support, limited postural sway
	Dynamic: Patient accepts *moderate challenge*; able to maintain balance while picking object off floor
Fair	**Static:** Patient able to maintain balance with handhold support; may require occasional *minimal assistance*
	Dynamic: Patient accepts *minimal challenge*; able to maintain balance while turning head/trunk
Poor	**Static:** Patient requires handhold support and moderate to *maximal assistance* to maintain position
	Dynamic: Patient unable to accept challenge or move without loss of balance

Adapted from O'Sullivan and Schmitz (1).

6. **Gait:** With technological assistance, the eight phases of gait can be reliably identified. They include: initial contact (IC), loading response (LR), midstance (MSt), terminal stance (TSt), preswing (PS), initial swing (ISw), midswing (MSw), and terminal swing (TSw). These can be further categorized into four phases: (1) weight acceptance (IC and LR), (2) stance (MSt and TSt), (3) forward progression (TSt and PS), and (4) swing (ISw, MSw,

and TSw). In an examination room without machines, identify if there were neuropathic gait abnormalities such as steppage gait, circumduction gait, Trendelenburg gait, or antalgic gait. If possible, gait should be examined indoors, outdoors, and on stairs.

Neurologic

1. **Cranial nerve (CN) testing**
   - **CN I (olfactory):** It may be helpful to carry a small plastic bottle that contains coffee, for example, and perform a simple bedside test to check the integrity of the sense of smell.
   - **CN II (optic), III (occulomotor), IV (trochlear), and VI (abducens)** are all related to the visual system.
   - **CN II (optic):** This can be evaluated via (1) Snellen charts with and without refractive lenses to test visual acuity, (2) Ishihara color dots to identify color blindness, (3) visual confrontation tests to identify any visual field defects, (4) light pens to check for direct and concentric papillary reflexes that also involves CN III as the efferent component, and (5) ophthalmoscope to check for the integrity of the optic fundus.
   - **CN III (occulomotor), IV (trochlear), and VI (abducens)** are typically tested together because coordinated extra-ocular movement in all directions depends on them for proper function. There is some overlap in their actions, summarized below:
     - **CN III (oculomotor)** innervates all other muscles in eye movements. It also raises eyelid and mediates pupilary constriction.
     - **CN VI (abducens)** innervates lateral rectus muscle, which moves eye laterally.

– **CN IV (trochlear)** innervates superior oblique muscle that moves eye downward and also rotates the eyeball internally.
- **CN V (trigeminal):** This nerve has both sensory and motor components. The sensory component covers 3 regions of the face: ophthalmic, maxillary, and mandibular. This can be tested by asking the patient to close his/her eyes, and then gently touching the areas while comparing side to side. The motor component innervates the temporalis and masseter muscles for mastication. This can be tested by asking the patient to clenches his/her jaws and grind his/her teeth, while the examiner palpates the above muscles.
- **Combination of CN V (sensory component of trigeminal) and VII (motor component of facial):** This can be tested by the corneal reflex. The examiner uses a piece of clean, soft cotton to touch the cornea (ophthalmic region of CN V), and observes the associated eyeblink, which is innervated by CN VII.
- **CN VII (facial):** The facial nerve innervates the muscles for facial expression, anterior 2/3 of the tongue's taste sense, as well as the stapedius muscle in the middle ear. The muscles innervated by facial nerve can be tested by asking the patient to (1) raise his/her eyebrows or frown (while examiner looks for forehead creases), (2) close the eyelids against resistance, (3) smile or show his/her teeth, and (4) puff out his/her cheeks. It is important to observe for facial symmetry. In supranuclear or upper motor neuron CN VII lesions, because of the inherent bilateral innervations of the upper facial muscles (frontalis and orbicularis oculi), weakness is only seen on the contralateral, lower facial muscles. In infranuclear or lower motor

neuron CN VII lesions such as Bell's palsy, both upper and lower facial weakness manifest on the side of the lesion. While stapedius muscle weakness may manifest as intolerance to sound (hyperacusis), taste sensation in the anterior 2/3 of the tongue can be easily tested by a sugar-coated lollipop or saline-dipped Q-tip.

- **CN VIII (auditory-vestibular or vestibular-cochlear nerve):** It works to transmit signals for hearing and equilibrium from the inner ear to the brain.

  - **Auditory component:** The examiner can stand behind the patient and present a ticking clock to the left and then the right ear, asking the patient if he/she can hear it. Without the clock, the examiner can simply rub the first and second fingers to create the sound. The Rinne test is also commonly used, by placing a vibrating tuning fork on the patient's mastoid process, and then next to the ear on the same side, to determine which of the two presentations was perceived as louder. A patient with normal hearing would find the latter to be louder.

  - **Vestibular component:** The doll's eye maneuver involves a rapid passive rotation of the head laterally. Normally, both eyes will move in a direction opposite the head rotation. Caloric testing is carried out most simply by irrigating the external auditory canal (observed by otoscope to be unobstructed by wax, not infected, and with no tympanic perforation) with water warmer or colder than body temperature, the presumed resting temperature of the labyrinths.

- **CN IX and X (glossopharyngeal and vagus nerves):** The function of these two nerves can be testing by the involuntary gag reflex. The soft palate should elevate when the examiner uses a tongue depressor to gently press against the posterior pharyngeal wall. This gives the examiner an idea of integrity of the sensory and motor components of CN IX and X. The motor components of CN IX and X can further be delineated by asking the patient to say "Ka" or "Ah." Normally the soft palate should elevate symmetrically. The uvula will deviate to the normal side. Though rarely done, the examiner can further test the sensory component of CN IX by introducing a bitter tasting solution to the posterior 1/3 and side of the tongue.

- **CN XI (accessory nerve):** CN XI innervates the trapezius and sternocleidomastoid muscles. The trapezius muscle can be tested by asking the patient to elevate or shrug his/her shoulders against resistance. The sternocleidomastoid muscle can be tested by asking the patient to turn the head against resistance, and observing the bulk of the muscle that is opposite to the direction of the head turn.

- **CN XII (hypoglossal nerve):** CN XII can be tested by asking the patient to protrude his/her tongue, and move it from left to right. If there is a unilateral lesion, the tongue will deviate toward the weak side.

2. **Deep tendon reflexes (DTRs)**

   A reflex hammer is typically used to elicit DTRs by sudden tapping to stretch the muscle and tendon. As in manual muscle testing, it is important to compare side to side for symmetry.

   - The commonly used scale to grade DTRs is as follows:
     - 0: Absent
     - 1^+: Trace
     - 2^+: Normal
     - 3^+: Brisk

- 4⁺: Nonsustained repetitive vibratory movements (clonus)
- 5⁺: Sustained clonus
- The commonly examined muscle-tendon groups and their corresponding root levels is listed as follows:
  - Biceps and brachioradialis: C5/C6
  - Triceps: C6/C7
  - Patellar: L2-L4
  - Ankle: S1

3. **Primitive reflexes (frontal release signs)**
   Adult patients with frontal lobe damage often demonstrate recurrence of infant like primitive reflexes such as the sucking reflex, rooting reflex, grasping reflex, and snout reflex. The sucking reflex refers to an infant's instinct to suck anything that touches the roof of his/her mouth. The rooting reflex refers to an infant's instinct to turn his/her head toward the side that the cheek that was being stroked. These reflexes were present to facilitate breastfeeding.
   - **Snout reflex:** This primitive reflex is often tested by light tapping of the closed lips near the midline, resulting in pursing of the lips.
   - **Glabellar (tap) reflex:** This is another primitive reflex. It is elicited by tapping on the forehead (afferent signal via the trigeminal nerve) of the patient, who typically responds by blinking (innervated by the facial nerve).
   - **Palmar grasp reflex:** This is also an infantile reflex that normally remains until 6 months old. When the examiner places an object in the infant's hand and strokes his/her palm, the infant's fingers will close to grasp the object.
   - **Brainstem reflexes:** These reflexes are involuntary responses to external stimuli mediated by the brainstem. Many brainstem reflexes involve the eyes either

as an area to stimulate, or as a location to observe for appropriate response. For example, when an examiner shines a bright light into one eye, both pupils should constrict. Other brainstem reflexes include coughing and gagging when the throat is irritated.

- **Oculocardiac reflex:** This reflex is due to connections between CN V (ophthalmic branch of the trigeminal nerve) and the parasympathetic nervous system through the vagus nerve (CN X). It manifests as bradycardia (decreased heart rate) in response to compression of the eyeball.

- **Horizontal oculocephalic reflex and oculovestibular reflex:** In the oculocephalic reflex, when the examiner turns the patient's head horizontally, the eyes should track in the opposite direction of the turn. In the oculovestibular reflex, the eyes move in the opposite direction to the side of the ear that is irrigated with cold water.

- **Pupillary light reflex:** When an examiner shines a bright light into one eye, both pupils should constrict, allowing less light to enter the fundus.

- **Vertical oculocephalic/oculovestibular reflex:** This reflex is meant to stabilize the incoming image and preserve it on the center of the visual field during head movement. It is accomplished by reflexive eye movement in the direction opposite to head movement. When the head is passively turned upward, the eyeballs will roll downward.

- **Fronto-orbicular reflex:** Just like the glabellar tap reflex, it is observed as contraction of the orbicularis oculi muscles in response to percussion of the frontal or forehead area (glabella).

- **Bowel reflex:** The lower bowels respond involuntarily to certain stimuli, such as movement after stretching of the stomach as a result of eating (gastrocolic reflex).

The intrinsic myenteric defecation reflex is the increase in peristalsis due to distension of the rectal wall. When the peristalsis arrives at the anus, the usually constricted internal anal sphincter will relax to allow stool passage.

- **Bladder reflex:** This is sometimes referred to as the micturition reflex. As the urine accumulates more in the bladder, stretching of the bladder wall causes afferent impulses to pass through the sacral region of the spinal cord, leading to firing of the parasympathetic efferent neurons that innervate the bladder's smooth muscles. This contraction further increases tension inside the bladder, causing further afferent input and resultant contraction, until the urine is emptied via relaxation of the sphincter muscles. If the sphincter does not relax in response to increasing bladder pressure, a condition called detrusor-sphincter dyssynergia occurs.

- **Cremasteric reflex:** This is a superficial reflex which is unique to males. When the medial and inner side of the thigh is gently stroked, an involuntary contraction of the cremasteric muscle occurs, pulling up the scrotum and the testicle in it. It is absent in complete spinal cord injury, some motor neuron diseases, and testicular torsion.

- **Bulbocavernosus reflex (BCR):** Unlike the cremasteric reflex, the BCR is normally present in both males and females. It can be elicited by stimulating the penis (squeezing the glans) or vulva (gently touching the lateral side of the clitoris with a cotton tip applicator) and observing contraction of the anal sphincter. This spinal mediated reflex is absent in spinal shock.

- **Anal wink reflex:** This is also referred to as the perineal reflex. It is similar to the BCR, except that the stimulus is stroking on the skin around the anus. The response is involuntary contraction of the anal sphincter muscle.

4. Cerebellar testing

This involves finger-to-nose test, heel-to-shin test, rapid alternating movement (RAM) test, and Romberg's test.

- **Finger-to-nose test (upper extremity dysmetria):** The examiner asks the patient to extend his/her arm first, followed by touching his/her nose, and then extend his/her arm to touch the examiner's finger. A positive result indicates upper extremity dysmetria.
- **Heel-to-shin test (lower extremity dysmetria):** The examiner asks the patient to rub his/her heel down the shin on the opposite side. If the patient is unable to keep his/her foot on the opposite shin, it indicates lower extremity dysmetria.
- **RAM:** The examiner asks the patient to place one of his/her hands over the other, and alternate the positions by flipping one of the hands on top and then at the bottom. If the patient is unable to perform this task in a smooth manner, it indicates dysdiadochokinesia.
- **Romberg's test:** The examiner stands near the patient to catch him/her in case of falls, and then asks the patient to stand with his eyes closed, without physical support from the examiner. The test is positive if the patient sways to either side or loses balance.
- **Fine and gross motor skills and coordination:** Fine motor skills include small muscle coordination to perform functions such as writing, twisting a pencil, moving the eyes, or moving the lips. Gross motor skills include walking, running, sitting, and pushing an object away. As the brain develops, the gross motor skills develop first, followed by gradual acquisition of fine motor skills.
- **Cerebellar tremor:** By definition, tremor is an involuntary oscillatory or rhythmic muscle movement. Cerebellar tremor can be elicited during a

finger-to-nose test. It is also called intention tremor because it manifests as a slow tremor that occurs at the end of a purposeful movement.

5. **Autonomic nervous system (ANS) testing**
   The ANS testing involves measurements of the heart rate, blood pressure, and also sweat function. These measurements should be taken at baseline, and in response to possible triggers. For example, a tilt table may be included and the above physiologic functional measures are recorded at different tilt angles. Sweat function hyperactivity can be observed with increases in skin humidity, or by connecting the patient to recording devices in a chamber. Heart rate and blood pressure can also be monitored in the chamber, although most clinics are not equipped to perform this on a regular basis.

General Medical Exam

1. **Skin:** Examination of the skin should include inspection of the hair, nails, and also the mucous membranes. This will give the examiner an overall picture of hydration and nutritional status of the patent. Causes of decreased skin turgor include: heat stroke (excessive sweating and decreased fluid input), diarrhea, vomiting, and excessive urination from poorly controlled diabetes. Hair and nails reveal the hygienic and nutritional status of the patient. In addition, tattoos may reveal the patient's religious belief or personal history, and often serves as a conversation opener for psychosocial history.

2. **Heart and circulation:** The examination begins with a general inspection of the skin/mucosal color and perfusion status, to find out if any pallor or cyanosis exists. This is usually followed by palpation for an arterial pulse

and measurement of blood pressure. The peripheral veins are inspected to rule out any distension or varicosity. The jugular vein should also be inspected and palpated. Percussion and palpation of the precordial region will give an approximation of heart location and movement. Auscultation is performed with a standard stethoscope, to identify the heart sounds (S1, S2), and murmurs. The murmurs can be categorized into (1) systolic versus diastolic, (2) continuous versus associated with a specific cardiac cycle, and (3) radiating versus localized. The quality and duration should also be described. If any chest tightness or pathological murmur is identified, a cardiology consultation will be needed.

3. **Lungs:** As in the examination of the heart and circulatory system, it is important to perform inspection, palpation, percussion, and auscultation of the lungs.
   - The first visual **inspection** will reveal if the patient has labored, distressed, or diaphoretic breathing. Normal breathing should be deep and regular. The use of accessory muscles such as sternocleidomastoids and scalene during breathing indicates dyspnea. Cyanosis around the lips and nail beds indicate poor oxygenation or hypoxemia.
   - On **palpation** of the posterior chest wall, the examiner can ask the patient to say "99," and feel a vibratory sensation during phonation. This normal vibratory sensation is called fremitus, which is reduced in pleural effusion.
   - **Percussion** of the lungs will produce a resonant sound. In pleural effusion or pneumonia, percussion will produce a dull sound.
   - **Auscultation:** There most common abnormal lung sounds are (1) *rales*: these are small bubbling or rat-

tling sounds that occur when closed air spaces are opened during air flow; (2) *rhonchi*: these low-pitched sounds occur when air flow overcomes resistance or blockage through a larger airway, making sounds that mimic snoring; (3) *wheezing*: these are sharp-pitched sounds that occur when airway is narrowed, like a whistling sound heard in lungs under asthma attack; and (4) *stridor*: these high-pitched, wheeze-like sounds occur due to a blockage of airflow in the posterior pharynx or trachea.

4. **Digestive system**

Examination of the digestive system begins with a **visual inspection** of the mouth and throat for ulcers, open lesions, and dental conditions that may affect solid food intake. Abdominal distension can be caused by intestinal obstruction (often associated with discomfort and restlessness), ascites (often accompanied by jaundice, distended shiny abdominal skin and everted umbilicus), or obesity (a round, soft belly with inverted umbilicus).

- **Palpation:** First, the examiner should ask the patient to identify any area that is painful or tender to touch. Since abdominal guarding may be misinterpreted as a hard mass, the examiner palpates the areas in question last, to give time for the patient to acclimatize to palpation and reduce "guarding" or "tensing."
- **Auscultation** of bowel sounds should be conducted with the diaphragm side of the stethoscope. The normal bowel sounds are intermittent, high frequency, gurgling, and clicking in nature, occurring about 10 times per minute. Peritonitis and neurogenic bowel obstruction often manifest with absent bowel sounds. Bruits are whooshing sounds that can be heard in abdominal aneurysm.

- **Percussion** is typically tympanic in nature, because in the supine position, air tends to rise to the anterior aspect of the abdominal cavity. Gaseous distension results in hyperresonance. A mass or fluid below the examined area will result in hyporesonance or dullness to percussion.
- Typically, after rapport has been established, examination of the digestive system concludes with inspection, palpation, or digital examination of the external rectal area to check for the presence of bleeding, hemorrhoids, or other suspicious masses.

5. **Genitourinary system:** If indicated, examination of the genitourinary system is typically reserved as the last part of the office visit, after the patient and physician have established sufficient rapport. The examiner should wear a glove during the process, and another health professional, preferably a registered nurse, should also be present. For a male patient, check for lesions on the genitals such as ulcers. Retract the foreskin if needed, to examine the glans and urethral orifice. Check for discharge. Though infrequently requested, the scrotum may be palpated to check for swelling and inflammation. For the female patient, check for superficial lesions, and note any discharge from the vaginal or urethral orifice. Unless requested, prostate and pelvic exams can be reserved for another same-day appointment with urology and gynecologist, respectively.

6. **Endocrine system:** Since the endocrine system affects the whole person in many ways, its bedside evaluation requires examination of the patient from head to toe, in a systemic manner, which is summarized as follows:

- **General appearance:** Height, weight, and any characteristic of stature that may suggest a syndrome. For example, patients with Cushing's syndrome often present with weight gain and moon face, which is due to fatty tissue deposits. Tall stature is typical in Marfan's syndrome, and short stature is common in hypothyroidism.
- **Blood pressure:** High for Cushing's syndrome; low for Addison's disease.
- **Hair:** In hypopituitarism, hair loss in the armpit is often noted.
- **Face:** Patients with Cushing's syndrome often have oily skin and acne, while patients with Marfan's syndrome tend to have an enlarged tongue and chin. Panhypopituitarism may present with hirsutism.
- **Eyes:** Protruding eyeballs or exophthalmos is typically seen in hyperthyroidism.
- **Mouth:** In Addison's disease, pigmentation in buccal mucosa can be easily visualized.
- **Neck:** Stand behind the patient and palpate the thyroid gland for goiter. In Cushing's syndrome, supraclavicular fat pads and buffalo hump are commonly observed. A webbed neck is seen in Turner's syndrome.
- **Hands:** Tremor, excessive warmth, and redness suggest hyperthyroidism. Oversized hands suggest acromegaly in Marfan's syndrome.
- **Chest:** While male gynecomastia is seen in Cushing's syndrome, reduced female breast size is observed in panhypopituitarism.
- **Abdomen:** Excessive abdominal fat and purple striae are seen in Cushing's syndrome.

- **Genitalia:** Regarding gonadal atrophy, it should be noted that prolonged administration of gonadal hormones actually reduces the production and output of gonadotropin from the pituitary gland, which may result in gonadal atrophy.
- **Lower extremities:** Patients with chronic diabetes mellitus often have peripheral neuropathy, and poor vascularization, which lead to diabetic foot ulcers.

In conclusion, because of the complicated feedback mechanisms involved, endocrine disorders often involve a combination of hyposecretion and hypersecretion of hormones, resulting in a mixed picture that requires complete laboratory work up and challenge tests. It is prudent to consult with an endocrinologist when the examination raises red flags for underlying endocrine abnormality or syndromes.

REFERENCE

1. O'Sullivan SB, Schmitz TJ. *Physical Rehabilitation: Assessment and Treatment*. 5th ed. Philadelphia, PA: F. A. Davis Company; 2007:254.

Ordering Tests

NEUROIMAGING

1. Initially after polytrauma, neuroimaging is used to assess for evidence of intracranial bleeding (CT scanning) or neuronal tissue injury of brain or spinal cord (MRI scanning). These modalities are utilized to determine the need for intensive care unit (ICU) monitoring/ management and surgical interventions.

2. Individuals with mild traumatic brain injury (mTBI)/concussion who rapidly (ie, within 30 minutes) return to their neurologic and symptomatic baseline (ie, are "normal") have no specific indication for neuroimaging. The goal of neuroimaging after concussion is to rule out significant, occult abnormalities (eg, subdural hematoma) that require more intensive care or monitoring, not to define the specific concussion-related pathology. While newer technologies have a higher sensitivity to detecting abnormalities after concussion, it is unclear whether or not they have any clinical relevance. Evidence of small amounts of subarachnoid

hemorrhage classify mTBIs as "complicated"; however, this has no specific clinical or prognostic significance.

3. Once medical and neurologic stability are achieved, repeat imaging of the brain or spinal cord is reserved for patients with poor recovery early ("plateauing" in first 2–6 weeks), any evidence of worsening, or with evidence of hydrocephalus on initial scanning. All individuals with a moderate to severe initial TBI who have not returned to baseline by 4 to 6 weeks postinjury and are being discharged from the hospital (acute or rehabilitation) should have a repeat brain CT scan to assess for hydrocephalus (or other rarer abnormality).

4. While neuroimaging can often be correlated with physiological deficits (in particular the newer, more precise techniques), in general it is not useful to use imaging to explain or identify physical, cognitive, behavioral, or functional deficits.

5. Neuroimaging has not demonstrated reliability in predicting clinically meaningful short- or long-term outcomes, although evidence of significant cerebral edema with compression (ie, shift of midline brain structures more than 5 mm) and large overall brain abnormalities (extensive "burden" of blood from multiple subdural, epidural, intraparenchymal, and subarachnoid injuries) seems to be associated with slower recovery.

6. As newer technologies (fMRI, PET, SPECT, HDFT) and techniques (DTI) emerge, there are increasing pressures to utilize additional neuroimaging to better understand persistent difficulties or symptoms; however, clinical practicality and validity are lacking.

NEUROPSYCHOLOGICAL EVALUATION

1. Neuropsychological testing is a general term to describe the standardized evaluations designed to assess cognitive

and behavioral functioning. The specifics and extent of testing used is typically tailored to the individual to be tested and the specific menu of tests selected may be related to a large number of factors, including presumed primary pathology, secondary medical and psychological conditions, acuity and severity of injury or insult, ability of patient to tolerate time and intensity of testing, cultural background and literacy of the patient, prior exposure to testing, training and experience of neuropsychologist, and goals of the evaluation. Only tests that have been shown to be valid and reliable measures for the conditions being considered should be utilized.

2. While neuropsychological testing may be administered and tabulated by any trained and certified examiner (psychometrist), interpretation should be restricted to a trained and certified neuropsychologist who is also aware of the examinee's history and physical findings. The use of "raw data" from neuropsychology testing to make diagnoses, base treatment, or define prognosis is invalid and inappropriate.

3. Neuropsychological testing may serve a number of functions and these should be identified in advance of the testing to allow the neuropsychologist to tailor the testing (type, extent, timing). While testing in isolation cannot be used to diagnose specific conditions (eg, concussion), they can be used by the patient's clinicians to support the overall diagnosis. More commonly, neuropsychological testing is used to define an individual's current cognitive and behavioral functioning, as well as the type, extent, and severity of any areas of abnormality. This can be used to establish a baseline, to identify areas of strength to take advantage of in therapy, to identify areas of weakness or deficit to help structure interventions (eg, therapy,

medication, education), to provide limitations (eg, no driving, no use of firearms), to identify adaptive strategies (eg, limiting complexity of tasks, optimize settings to enhance attention), and to monitor changes over time. Optimally, the patient's clinicians will work closely with the neuropsychologist to determine the best timing for and specific tests to be used ("Why is testing being requested?," "What questions are you looking to answer?") and to make use of the information found.

4. Given the learning that can occur with repeated testing, most neuropsychological measures should not be repeated (if being used for testing purposes) any more often than annually. A sample battery of brief tests that are appropriate for individuals with TBI might include:

- **NIH Toolbox Cognition Battery**. The NIH Toolbox is a recently developed comprehensive assessment tool with an emphasis on measuring outcomes in longitudinal epidemiologic studies and prevention or intervention trials across the lifespan. The cognition battery is a brief and efficient computer-based neuropsychological test of the 7 key cognitive domains: Executive Function, Episodic Memory, Working Memory, Processing Speed, Language, Attention, and Reading. The full battery requires only 20 to 30 minutes to administer.

- **Continuous Performance Test (CPT).** The CPT is a classic sustained attention response inhibition task that requires subjects to respond to a certain type of stimulus and withhold a response to another. The "examiner version" is specifically reliable and valid to assess executive function across a wide range of ages and disorders. It takes 4 to 5 minutes to complete.

- **Working Memory Index (Digit Span, Letter-Number Sequencing) and Processing Speed Index (Symbol**

Search, Coding) subtests of the Wechsler Adult Intelligence Scale, 4th Version (WAIS-IV). The WAIS-IV is one of the most established and commonly used instruments for the assessment of IQ. Administration time for WAIS-IV subtests is about 20 minutes.

- **Trail Making Test (TMT) Parts A and B.** The TMT is a test of visual attention and task switching. The TMT requires visuomotor integration while engaging in concurrent mental manipulation of numbers and letters and thus provides a measure of executive control. It can provide information about visual search speed, scanning, speed of processing, mental flexibility, and executive functioning. It is also sensitive to detecting several cognitive impairments such as Alzheimer's disease and dementia. The test requires 2 to 10 minutes, depending on degree of impairment.

- **Delis-Kaplan Executive Function System (D-KEFS) Color-Word Interference Test** (also known as the Stroop Test). Originally designed by Stroop, it is the most widely used clinical test of inhibition. The color-word interference condition is the primary measure of inhibition and involves the suppression of the prepotent response to read the word, rather than name the color of the word. The DKEFS version of the Stroop has the advantage of using the color and word reading conditions as controls for the interference and switching conditions.

- **Rey Auditory Verbal Learning Test (RAVLT) (Three Trial Version).** The RAVLT evaluates a wide diversity of cognitive functions: verbal learning and memory including retroactive and proactive interference, retention, in-coding versus retrieval, and subjective organization. Approximately 10 to 15 minutes is required.

- **Brief Visuospatial Memory Test-Revised (BVMT-R).** The BVMT-R is a measure of immediate and delayed visual memory. The test requires 10 minutes to administer.
- **Delis-Kaplan Executive Function System (D-KEFS) Verbal Fluency Test (VFT).** The VFT is composed of three conditions: letter fluency (aka the Controlled Oral Word Association Test), category fluency, and category switching. It measures an individual's ability to generate words fluently in an effortful, phonemic format, from overlearned concepts, while simultaneously shifting between these concepts. It requires 6 minutes to administer.

II

Diagnosis and

Management of

Common Sequelae

of Traumatic Brain Injury

5

Focal Weakness and Hypotonia

1. Following polytrauma, focal weakness of a limb or side of the body may occur from central (brain, spinal cord) or peripheral (plexus, nerve, muscle, joint) cause. Identifying the cause(s) of the weakness is useful in recommending therapeutic interventions and in prognosticating outcome.

2. The presence of hypotonia (a decrease in the resting tension) in a muscle, usually accompanied by a decrease or loss of deep tendon reflexes in the affected region, is most often seen with a neurologic etiology of injury. Acutely, both upper (brain, spinal cord) and lower (plexus, nerve) motor neuron injuries will result in hypotonia; however, chronically (after 6 weeks), upper motor neuron (UMN) injuries usually manifest with hypertonia, spasticity, or a return to normal tone. A true decrease in muscle tone (and reflexes) after injury or insult is typically diagnostic of a persistent abnormality of a peripheral nerve

(whether at the anterior horn cell/plexus origin or more distal). Given the complexity of many polytrauma injuries, it is important to be aware that some individuals may have both upper and lower motor neuron (LMN) injuries with variable findings in different parts of either the body or even the same limb.

3. Limb (muscle) weakness caused by focal trauma or insult to a muscle or joint, with or without pain, will typically resolve relatively rapidly (within 6 weeks) with a gradated program of general functional activity. Often there is deconditioning weakness related to a decrease in use. Focal strengthening of the affected region can also be utilized, often accompanied by pain management (thermal, tactile and electrical modalities, medications) techniques.

4. Limb weakness caused by a LMN injury or insult will often take considerably longer to improve and may not fully recover if the peripheral nerve abnormality persists (ie, the nerve does not fully heal). Muscle atrophy, which is often first noticed as a "prominence" of the underlying boney structures, is common with incomplete nerve recovery. Joints with atrophied and chronically weakened muscles are at an elevated risk for subluxation, dislocation, and long-term arthritic changes. Regular and frequent controlled stretching and positioning is performed to maintain the flexibility of the structures (muscle, tendon, ligament, joint) involved. Oftentimes, a splint may be required to maintain the foundation of the region and for protection. Gradated strengthening and functional tasking (eg, walking, dressing) should be performed

frequently throughout the day to optimize recovery by enhancing strength and coordination. Caution must always be taken in individuals who have a loss of sensation (often seen with LMN injury), with a specific focus on regular examination of the skin and a heightened safety awareness of the limb(s).

5. Limb weakness caused by UMN injury or insult may be approached in similar ways as LMN weakness, however it is more commonly associated with "hyperreactive" muscles (hypertonia, spasticity) that may make strengthening, coordination, and functional training more difficult. While atrophy is less common (the muscles may in fact hypertrophy from constant activation), shortening of the muscles with contractures of the joints where the muscles act is frequently a challenge. A rigorous program of relaxation, stretching, positioning, and carefully controlled activation is vital. Oftentimes, interventions to decrease tone (and actually initially further weaken the muscles) must also be utilized.

6. The use of functional electrical stimulation (FES) in persistent focal weakness, whether due to LMN or UMN insult, is common but of unclear long-term functional benefit due to the inconvenience, cost, and unclear efficacy. FES provides focused and intermittent electrical stimulation to either nerves or muscles to activate the affected muscle(s) and provide functional movement. FES is typically delivered via surface electrodes/pads from a Smartphone-sized stimulator. Newer systems that incorporate FES into orthoses (braces) or are implanted under the skin show promise.

Focal Weakness

Assessment

Focal weakness of a limb or side of the body may occur from either central or peripheral origin.

Identifying the cause(s) of the weakness is useful in recommending therapeutic interventions and in prognosticating outcome.

Precautions

The use of functional electrical stimulation (FES) in persistent focal weakness, whether due to lower motor neuron (LMN) or upper motor neuron (UMN) insult is common, but of unclear long-term functional benefit due to the inconvenience, cost, and unclear efficacy.

Caution must always be taken in individuals who have a loss of sensation (often seen with LMN injury), with a specific focus on regular examination of the skin and a heightened safety awareness of the limb(s).

Management

Limb (muscle) weakness caused by focal trauma or insult to a muscle or joint, with or without pain, will typically resolve relatively rapidly (within 6 weeks) with a gradated program of general functional activity.

Limb (nerve) weakness caused by a LMN injury or insult will often take considerably longer to improve and may not fully recover if the peripheral nerve abnormality persists (ie, the nerve does not fully heal).

Limb weakness caused by UMN injury or insult may be approached in similar ways as LMN weakness; however, it is more commonly associated with "hyperreactive" muscles (hypertonia, spasticity) that may make strengthening, coordination, and functional training more difficult.

Treatment focused on stretching, positioning, gradated strengthening, and the application of adaptive aids for safety and function.

6

Spasticity

1. Following polytrauma, individuals with upper motor neuron (UMN; brain, spinal cord) injury or insult will commonly have weakness of the limbs and the part of the body controlled by the injured region. While for the first several days to weeks after injury, the resting muscle tone or tone with movement may be normal or decreased, usually there will be an increase in the resting tone (hypertonia), reflexes (hyperreflexia), and resistance to movement (spasticity). While these difficulties may resolve as the central nervous system (CNS) abnormality improves, it is vital to optimize recovery and function of the affected limb or body region whether full recovery occurs or not. The more severe the initial injury (brain or spinal cord), the more likely there will be focal areas of spasticity that will persist for longer periods of time. Typically the antigravity muscles of flexion of the limbs and trunk are most affected. The 5-point modified Ashworth Scale (MAS) is the most commonly used metric to quantify the degree and functional impact of limb spasticity.

2. While spasticity can occur in the trunk and back region (and even the bladder), most commonly with spinal cord injuries (usually affecting the cervical cord), it is important to differentiate spastic muscles from muscles in "spasm." Muscle spasms are focal phenomenon of unclear etiology and pathophysiology that occur in neurologically intact individuals when muscles are acutely or chronically overused or stressed. They can also accompany general physical or psychological stress. They have no relationship to the "neurologic spasticity" seen after UMN, although they can occur in individuals with UMN. Importantly, they should be managed with local modalities (heat, ice, massage), stretching, and gradated return to active usage, along with general strategies to enhance overall conditioning, relaxation and stress management, and good sleep hygiene.

3. Limb spasticity, with accompanying weakness and functional loss, caused by UMN injury or insult must combine techniques to decrease the tone/spasticity with limb retraining, strengthening, and enhancing coordination. Regular and frequent controlled stretching and positioning is performed to maintain the flexibility of the structures (muscle, tendon, ligament, joint) involved. Oftentimes, a splint may be required to maintain the maximal range of motion (ROM). Gradated strengthening and functional tasking (eg, walking, dressing) should be performed frequently throughout the day to optimize recovery by enhancing strength and coordination.

4. Interventions to decrease hypertonia/spasticity must be implemented early (within the first week of identification) and increased in intensity if the results are limited to prevent a loss of ROM to decrease pain and to prevent a cycle of increasing spasticity brought on by the

noxious stimuli of pain and forced stretch. Initial interventions focus on decreasing noxious stimuli (pain, swelling, infection, tight clothing, intravenous needles, wounds, or pressure sores), several times daily ROM and proper positioning, and frequent surveillance. If spasticity persists (and thus limb movement and use is decreased or prevented), tactile, thermal, and electrical modalities are used to stimulate local and central pathways. Oral antispasmodics may be used if these modalities are not fully successful in the first week of usage; however, they are best suited for multilimb (hemibody or full body) spasticity. Focal persistence of spasticity of the arm or leg that is limiting joint ROM, is painful, or is preventing functional movement of the limb for more than 2 weeks should be managed with intraneuronal (eg, phenol) or intramuscular neurolytics (eg, botulinum toxin). While a common effect of these treatments is initial weakening of the involved muscles, the marked reduction seen in spasticity is far more important. Gradated strengthening and coordination exercises may be implemented as soon as the spasticity is improved. Combining the systemic effects of oral antispasmodics with the focal effect of a neurolytic is the best approach for multilimb spasticity.

5. To decrease multilimb spasticity that is affecting ROM, causing significant pain, or limiting functional recovery, oral antispasmodics are often needed. While dantrolene sodium (25–100 mg 2–4 times daily) is the recommended first-line agent because of its non sedating peripheral location of action (ie, calcium channel blockade), the need for an extremely slow dosing program and limited actual effects limit its practical usage. Lioresal (10–40 mg 2–4 times daily) is typically the most effective

agent and its central sedating or cognitively impairing side effects tend to well tolerated.

6. The use of functional electrical stimulation (FES) in persistent focal weakness or incoordination with UMN insult is common, but of unclear long-term functional benefit due to the inconvenience, cost, and unclear efficacy. FES provides focused and intermittent electrical stimulation to either nerves or muscles to activate the affected muscle(s) and provide functional movement. FES is typically delivered via surface electrodes/pads from a Smartphone-sized stimulator. Newer systems that incorporate FES into orthoses (braces) or are implanted under the skin show promise.

Spasticity

Assessment

The modified Ashworth Scale is most commonly used to quantify the degree and functional impact of limb spasticity.

Precautions

Muscle spasms are focal phenomenon of unclear etiology and pathophysiology that can occur in neurologically intact individuals when muscles are acutely or chronically overused or stressed.

Management

Spasticity interventions must be implemented early and increased in intensity if the results are limited to prevent a loss of range of motion, to decrease pain and to prevent a cycle of increasing spasticity brought on by the noxious stimuli of pain and forced stretch.

Initial interventions focus on decreasing noxious stimuli, range of motion several times daily, proper positioning, and frequent surveillance.

If spasticity persists, then tactile, thermal, and electrical modalities are used to stimulate local and central pathways.

Oral antispasmodics may be used if these modalities are not fully successful in the first week of usage; however, they are best suited for multilimb spasticity.

Focal persistence of spasticity of the arm or leg that is limiting joint range of motion, is painful, or is preventing functional movement of the limb for more than 2 weeks should be managed with intraneuronal or intramuscular neurolytics.

7

Coordination and

Balance Deficits

1. Coordination involves a combination of body movements created with the kinematic and kinetic parameters that result in intended actions. Deficits after polytrauma may be the cause of either central (brain, spinal cord) or peripheral (nerve, muscle) difficulties, which result in problems with coordination. Injuries to the brain may produce generalized problems with coordination (cerebellum, basal ganglia) that can affect individual limbs (dysmetria) or the trunk (ataxia) or produce whole body perturbations (generalized ataxia). Injuries to the brain, spinal cord, nerves, or muscles may produce focal areas of weakness that manifest in coordination difficulties. Additionally, abnormalities in sensation of the limbs from damage or insult to the nervous system may manifest with coordination deficits. Finally, damage to either the brainstem or to the inner ear structures (labyrinthian system) of balance may result in difficulties with equilibrium and balance that manifest as coordination

deficits with dizziness (an impairment in spatial perception and stability).

2. Difficulties with dysmetria and weakness-related coordination problems will often respond to repeated controlled movements, strengthening and optimizing limb positioning for tasks, along with the natural recovery of injury. Importantly, slow and meticulous movements that accurately pattern the desired movement are key to improvement ("perfect practice makes perfect"). Weighted, oversized, and adaptive devices (eg, utensils, cups, razors) may serve both a therapeutic and functional purpose. A small number of patients may respond to tactile (wrist or ankle weights), auditory (bells on wrist), visual (the use of a mirror during tasks), and electrical (the use of low-level electrical stimulation during tasks) stimulation to improve limb coordination deficits. There are no specific braces that have clear benefit for limb dysmetria.

3. Truncal ataxia may be treated in a similar manner as limb dysmetria or weakness. Given the large number of muscles, nerve pathways, and factors (eg, sitting vs. standing, weight of body, support structures in sitting) affecting the trunk, however, recovery from or adaptation to ataxia is more difficult. The use of adaptive aids for sitting (eg, wheelchair, molded seat) and walking (walker, crutches) is often required and should be utilized early in the course of recovery. Truncal braces or supports have no role in ataxia and are likely to cause harm. Similarly, medications have not been shown to have any positive effect.

4. Balance deficits related to brainstem/labyrinthian structure injury or disorders (eg, Meniere's syndrome) do not result in difficulties in specifically coordinating the

trunk, but rather in an inability to maintain upright and other sustained functional positions of the head due to dizziness, nausea, and related discomfort. While these balance deficits may resolve spontaneously, more often strategies similar to those used for coordination deficits (gradated and repeated activity) are effective. Special attention is paid to neck and head range of motion, eye tracking and motion, and the integrity of the extremity and truncal proprioceptive system. Some patients respond favorably to alternating positioning of the head and neck while being rapidly and repeatedly taken from the seated to lying down position (known as the Liberatory technique or the Hallpike–Dix maneuver). While some clinicians advocate the usage of low-dose benzodiazepines to lower the threshold for vertigo (a subtype of dizziness in which a patient inappropriately experiences the perception of motion, usually spinning) and nausea, this must be weighed against the risks of sedation, confusion, falls, and addiction.

5. Balance deficits can be quantified with a number of standardized measures. The most commonly used following polytrauma are either the Berg Balance Scale (BBS) or computerized posturography (CPT). The BBS is made up of 14 actions that an examiner asks a patient to perform, rated 1 to 4, with a score of 56 being perfect. CPT utilizes a moveable force plate combined with variable visual stimuli to take the patient through a series of maneuvers that test the visual, proprioceptive, and vestibular systems. A third measure that is utilized, particularly with older adults, is the Timed Get Up and Go Test, which assesses an individual's ability to arise from sitting, walk 3 m, turn around, and return to the chair.

Coordination and Balance Deficits

Assessment

The Berg Balance Scale (BBS) is the gold standard physical assessment for balance after polytrauma.

Computerized posturography (CPT) provides an objective, validated, neurophysiologic assessment of balance.

The Timed Get Up and Go Test is a simple physical assessment of balance and gait.

Precautions

Balance and coordination deficits from polytrauma result from motor, sensory, vision, labyrinthian, and cognitive difficulties, so the approach must be multimodal.

Management

Repeated controlled movements, strengthening exercises, and optimizing limb positioning for tasks.

Slow and meticulous movements that accurately pattern the desired movement are essential to improvement ("perfect practice makes perfect").

Weighted, oversized, and adaptive devices may serve both a therapeutic and functional purpose.

Tactile, auditory, visual and electrical stimulation to improve limb coordination deficits may also help. There are no specific braces that have clear benefit.

The Liberatory technique or the Hallpike–Dix maneuver, alternating positioning of the head and neck while being rapidly and repeatedly taken from the seated to lying down position, may be rapidly effective.

Some clinicians advocate the usage of low-dose benzodiazepines to lower the threshold for vertigo.

8

Tremors

1. Tremors are rare manifestations of injury or insult to the brain from polytrauma. The presence of a new tremor from a brain abnormality signifies problems with the basal ganglia. Tremor represents one manifestation of the parkinsonism that can occur from these injuries and most commonly affects the upper extremities. Multilimb or truncal tremors are rare, but can be seen in very severe traumatic brain injury (TBI), especially in individuals with long periods of disorders of consciousness (coma). Other sources of tremor that the clinician must be aware of include extremity coordination (dysmetria) deficits from cerebellar abnormality, extremity shaking related to anxiety or substance use withdrawal (delirium tremons), or a preexisting condition. The most common causes of noninjury-related tremor include essential tremor (ET) and Parkinson's disease (PD).

2. While many of the interventions that are used to improve general coordination and weakness deficits of the extremities (eg, repeated controlled movements, strengthening,

and optimizing limb positioning for tasks) are often utilized for injury related tremors, they are rarely effective. Similarly, medications that target the basal ganglion structures linked to PD (the substantia nigra) or that may have an effect on ET are often utilized, but these also are rarely effective. Weighted, oversized, and adaptive devices (eg, utensils, cups, razors) may serve both a therapeutic and functional purpose. There are no specific braces that have clear benefit from tremors.

Dysphagia

1. Dysphagia is defined as difficulty swallowing and is frequently seen after any upper or lower motor neuron disorder affecting the brain. It is most commonly seen with injury or insult to the brainstem and alterations in any or all of the three phases (oral motor, pharyngeal, esophageal) of swallowing may be seen.

2. Until appropriate diagnostic evaluation can be performed, all patients should be placed on a strict nothing per oral (NPO) status who have a diagnosis of dysphagia or who have significant risk factors for dysphagia, including history of stroke, moderate/severe traumatic brain injury (TBI), altered mental status, history of aspiration, pneumonia, dysarthria, dysphonia, prolonged intubation, facial droop, tongue weakness or deviation upon protrusion, uvular deviation with sustained "ah," buccal pocketing of food, hypernasality, abnormal gag reflex, cough after swallowing, abnormal cough, wet vocal quality after swallowing, difficulty managing secretions, drooling.

3. A preliminary assessment step may be a bedside swallowing evaluation by a skilled speech-language pathologist or

physiatrist, but it is recommended that this be confirmed with a videofluorographic swallow study (VSS), also known as a modified barium swallow (MBS), which allows for visualization and assessment of all three stages of the swallow. Alternatively, flexible endoscopic evaluation of swallowing (FEES) may be performed but is less commonly employed because it does not allow observation of the pharyngeal stage of swallowing.

4. While some centers advocate the use of a Free Water Test (using 50 cc of sterile water) to determine the ability to swallow, the research supporting both its safety and its validity are scant.

5. The results of the MBS may be directly translated into a modified per oral (PO) diet:
   - National dysphagia diet levels:
     - Level 1: Pureed food (pudding-like consistency)
     - Level 2: Foods that are moist, soft, and easily formed into a bolus
     - Level 3: No hard, sticky, or crunchy foods
   - Thickened liquid consistencies:
     - Nectar/syrup
     - Honey
     - Pudding

6. Upgrading of diet frequently occurs over the days and weeks following the initial evaluation, under the guidance of a speech-language pathologist and ideally with a repeat MBS or FEES.

7. If thin liquids cannot be tolerated by 3 weeks postonset, a percutaneous endoscopic gastrostomy (PEG) tube should be placed. The PEG allows for efficient enteral hydration and nutrition while dysphagia therapy is ongoing. Even if swallowing skills recover rapidly, the

PEG tube must remain in place for at least 6 weeks to prevent formation of a gastrocutaneous fistula. PEG tubes must be examined daily and rotated one-quarter turn (90 degrees) daily to optimize skin integrity. PEG site irritation or cellulitis should be treated with a broad-spectrum oral antibiotic, such as Keflex, and a topical agent, such as Bacitracin.

8. Traditional swallowing therapy includes resistance exercises for the lips, jaw, and tongue; thermal-tactile stimulation of the facial arches to trigger swallowing; effortful swallowing and production of sustained high-pitched "ee" to promote laryngeal elevation; and hard glottal attack or Valsalva to promote vocal fold adduction. Although efficacy data are equivocal, some dysphagia therapists utilize neuromuscular electrical stimulation (NMES) of the laryngeal strap muscles at 1 to 25 milliamps (current increased until patient is able to generate audible swallow) during practice swallowing of safe consistencies.

9. Compensatory strategies for dysphagia include: chin tuck to prevent premature spillage in patients with poor bolus control; head turn to weak side, directing bolus toward strong side, for unilateral pharyngeal/laryngeal; head tilt toward strong side for unilateral oral weakness; supraglottic swallow (holding breath prior to swallow to improve laryngeal closure and coughing afterward to clear laryngeal residue); effortful swallow or double swallow to clear pharyngeal residue; Mendelsohn maneuver (hold larynx in elevated position during swallow) to help open the upper esophageal sphincter); and use of a palatal lift appliance to prevent nasal regurgitation of the bolus.

10. For patients with low aspiration risk but slow progress toward full oral hydration or nutrition due to altered

cognition, decreased arousal, or poor endurance, calorie and fluid counts should be obtained to ensure adequate nutrition and hydration. For patients under significant metabolic stress, the American Society for Parenteral and Enteral Nutrition guidelines indicate that carbohydrates should supply 50%–60% of total daily energy requirements, protein 20%–25% (approximately 1.5–2 g/kg/d), and fat 10%–30% of daily requirements.

11. For patients requiring long-term or permanent nonoral feeding, a long-term PEG tube, gastrojejunostomy tube, or jejunostomy tube may be needed. For tubes that terminate in the stomach, bolus feedings through large bore syringes are convenient for use at home and allow approximation of normal meal patterns but may not be tolerated due to rapid administration. Gravity drip feeding systems are available and allow for more protracted delivery of the product but are more expensive. Patients with jejunostomy tubes rarely tolerate bolus and gravity drip delivery, necessitating use of a feeding pump for controlled delivery.

Dysphagia

Assessment

A preliminary assessment step may be a bedside swallowing evaluation by a skilled speech-language pathologist or physiatrist, but it is recommended that this be confirmed with a videofluorographic swallow study (VSS) or modified barium swallow (MBS).

The VSS MBS allows for visualization and assessment of all three stages of the swallowing process.

Precautions

All patients with elevated risk or any evidence of dysphagia should be placed on a strict nothing per oral (NPO) until they can be evaluated by a speech and language pathologist.

Management

Dietary modifications based on MBS and placement of an enteral tube, as needed, to maintain nutrition and hydration are key first steps.

Swallowing therapy includes resistance exercises for the lips, jaw, and tongue; thermal stimulation of the facial arches to trigger swallowing; effortful swallowing and production of sustained "ee" to promote laryngeal elevation; and hard glottal attack or Valsalva to promote vocal fold adduction.

Neuromuscular electrical stimulation of the laryngeal strap muscles during practice swallowing of safe consistencies is also utilized.

Compensatory strategies focus on optimizing bolus formation and mobilization without spilling, pocketing, or overwhelming the impaired swallowing mechanism.

Numbness

1. Following polytrauma, a decrease (hypoesthesia) or complete loss (anesthesia) of sensation of a limb or side of the body may occur from a central (brain, spinal cord) or peripheral (nerve) cause. In addition to the sensation of numbness, the alteration in feeling may also be perceived as painful (dysesthesia). While most patients with numbness describe their limbs as being asleep or tingling, some may actually complain that their hands or feet feel "swollen." A side-to-side comparison between the involved and unaffected sides may be needed in the face of partial or slight injury. Weakness of the muscles supplied by the injured central or peripheral nerves is also common. Identifying the cause(s) of the numbness is useful in recommending therapeutic interventions and in prognosticating outcome.

2. Sensory deficits resulting from upper motor neuron (UMN) injury typically affect large portions of the body. When numbness results from brain injuries (usually from severe traumatic brain injury [TBI] with injury to the frontal cortex,

thalamus), it is most commonly near complete anesthesia affecting the contralateral arm and leg. Individuals with injury or insult to the thalamus typically have significant dysesthesia. Numbness from spinal cord injury is typically from the "level of injury" distal with partial loss in some areas around the injury ("zone of injury") and complete at the more distal aspects. Dysesthesias are not uncommon at these zones of injury. Lower motor neuron (LMN) injuries resulting from single or multiple peripheral nerve injury result in patchy deficits limited to the "neurotome" of that specific nerve. The degree of completeness of deficits is related to the severity of the injury (eg, bruised nerve versus transection). Partial injuries are more likely to result in some degree of dysesthesia as well. Given the complexity of many polytrauma injuries, it is important to be aware that some individuals may have both upper and LMN injuries with variable findings in different parts of the body or even the same limb.

3. There are no proven or commonly used interventions to specifically enhance recovery of sensation after central or peripheral nerve injury. Natural recovery (usually within 3–6 months) of sensory deficits is common after both UMN and LMN injuries, with greatest recovery in incomplete or milder injuries. Management is focused on optimizing overall health and medical conditions, education on avoidance of things that may delay or prevent recovery (smoking, alcohol use, neurotoxic medications or environmental exposures, repeat brain injury, repetitive trauma, or irritation of peripheral nerves). Additionally, caution must always be taken in individuals who have a loss of sensation, with a specific focus on regular examination of the skin and a heightened safety awareness of the affected limb (eg, monitoring for unnoticed cuts or abrasions, inadvertent burning on the stove).

Numbness

Assessment

Following polytrauma, a decrease (hypoesthesia) or complete loss (anesthesia) of sensation of a limb or a side of the body may occur from a central (brain, spinal cord) or peripheral (nerve) cause.

In addition to the sensation of numbness, sometimes an ordinary stimulus may be perceived as painful or unpleasant (dysesthesia).

A side-to-side comparison between the involved and unaffected sides may be needed in partial or slight injury.

Precautions

While most patients with numbness describe their limbs as being asleep or tingling, some may actually complain that their hands or feet feel "swollen." Always examine and compare bilaterally.

Management

There are no proven or commonly used interventions to specifically enhance recovery of sensation after central or peripheral nerve injury.

Management is focused on optimizing overall health and medical conditions, education on avoidance of things that may delay or prevent recovery (smoking, alcohol use, neurotoxic medications or environmental exposures, repeat brain injury, repetitive trauma, or irritation of peripheral nerves).

Caution must always be taken in individuals who have a loss of sensation, with a specific focus on regular examination of the skin and a heightened safety awareness of the affected limb (eg, monitoring for unnoticed cuts or abrasions, inadvertent burning on the stove).

11

Pain

1. Pain following polytrauma is common and typically multifactorial, with neurologic, psychologic, musculoskeletal, and iatrogenic etiologies. Improvement and resolution of pain symptoms are usually rapid (within 2–6 weeks) and often accompany mobilization and a return to activity. While medication use is commonly required in the first several weeks to allow for reactivation, this should be limited to nonopioid agents (eg, acetaminophen 500–1000 mg 3–4 times daily) that are used in a scheduled and at therapeutic levels. Judicious use of short-acting opioids are dispensed based on standardized pain scale monitoring (eg, Visual Analog Pain scale) for breakthrough pain. There is no role for ongoing use of either short- or long-acting opioid narcotics after the first 6 weeks.

2. Nonheadache pain related to an upper motor neuron (UMN; brain or spinal cord) injury is not typical, unless there is a focal injury to the thalamus. Thalamic pain is typically severe and allodynic (pain due to a stimulus that

does not normally provoke pain) in nature. While some patients benefit from the commonly used neuropathic pain agents (tricyclic antidepressants [TCAs], selective serotoninergic reuptake inhibitors [SSRIs]) or transcutaneous electrical nerve stimulation (TENS), this pain is typically intractable to treatment. Pain management techniques, such as relaxation training, biofeedback, and the use of visual imagery, that stress functioning despite the discomfort may be the best approach to optimize outcome. The dysesthetic or allodynic pain that may be seen around the zone of injury (especially in the shoulders of quadriplegics) after spinal cord injury is more likely the result of the lower motor neuron (LMN; peripheral nerve) and musculoskeletal injury and dysfunction seen with these injuries.

3. The pain associated with LMN injuries resulting from single or multiple peripheral nerve injury is usually dysesthetic in nature and limited to the "neurotome" of that specific nerve(s). Partial nerve injuries are more likely to result in some degree of dysesthesia, and some pain component is usually noted as these nerves recover (sprout or "regrow"). While a number of modalities (eg, thermal, tapping, vibration, compressive wraps) may provide temporary relief, both oral (atypical antidepressants, TCAs, SSRIs) and local (Capsaicin gel) neuropathic pain agents, and TENS are usually the most beneficial. Additionally, progressive return to meaningful physical activity and functional tasks will decrease pain. Optimizing overall health, nerve health (avoiding smoking, alcohol use, neurotoxic medications, environmental exposures, repetitive trauma, or irritation of peripheral nerves) and managing comorbid medical conditions are also an integral part of care.

4. Musculoskeletal causes of pain are manifold following polytrauma and the urgent surgical care often required. As noted, the majority of these injuries will recover within 2–6 weeks using a gradated program of activity and focal exercise (eg, stretching, strengthening, motor reeducation, coordination). Scheduled medications to reduce inflammation (often contraindicated acutely following fracture) and pain are usually utilized in this initial period, but care must be taken to wean off all medications as rapidly as possible. A rapid return to full weight-bearing, walking, and even fitness activities will not only enhance functional outcomes but also will decrease pain and psychological issues.

5. Psychological factors are common causes and contributors of pain following polytrauma. Many psychologic disorders, including posttraumatic stress disorder (PTSD) and depression, may manifest with focal or diffuse pain, which may be confused with neurologic or musculoskeletal injury. Fibromyalgia is a common example of this in the nontraumatic population. In addition to appropriate treatment of these psychological conditions (counseling, medications), the rapid physical remobilization, management of insomnia, and a focus on meaningful functional activities will be beneficial for both the pain and psychological conditions.

12

Vision Deficits

1. While vision deficits following polytrauma are relatively uncommon, their potential impact on a wide range of functional activities is so significant that all patients should be carefully evaluated to rule them out. The processing of visual signals by the brain and the understanding of the meaning of those signals by the cognitively impaired patient is more often the challenge seen ("central visual processing"). Oftentimes the patients with the highest chance of having vision deficits are those with the most severe brain dysfunction, which limits careful evaluation as well as the implementation of some of the adaptive and therapeutic strategies available. Individuals with mild traumatic brain injury (TBI) not uncommonly report double vision (diplopia) and light sensitivity (photophobia); however, these findings are usually self-limited and rarely directly impact vision. Difficulties with lateral gaze and pupillary tracking that cause challenges with visual scanning (including reading) may actually be a commonly

occurring problem after TBI (including concussion); however, it has not been well researched.

2. Visual acuity is not typically affected by brain injury, as it is related to the functioning of the eye itself. Brain dysfunction may cause a partial loss of visual fields (homonymous hemianopsia) and these are often not noted by the patient. Natural recovery is common by 3 months postinjury, but if recovery is poor, adaptive techniques ("lighthouse technique" of complete scanning of any new room) and eyewear (orthoptics, eg, Fresnel lenses) may be helpful.

3. Diplopia is essentially an incoordination of the visual signal by the brain resulting in out of phase images that are perceived as double. While there is no research to support the specific therapeutic value of eye "patching" on recovery rate, it is an excellent symptomatic relief for the patient (for both the double vision and the headaches often associated with it). Either eye may be "patched," but most clinicians advocate alternating the patching between eyes and having periods of time without patching. A better intervention than a patch is actually the use of translucent tape over one side of a pair of glasses (corrective or cosmetic) or a translucent patch. The translucency prevents the double vision, but also allows for light to pass to the eye, which is better tolerated and "normal" feeling.

4. Photophobia may be considered as a type of dysesthetic pain, which can quickly develop into a psychological condition (with concomitant pain behaviors). As with all painful conditions, it should be treated acutely (first 2–4 weeks) with "pain blocking agents" that are progressively weaned away as the patient is returned to full activity. In the case of photophobia, the blocking agents are not scheduled pain medication, but dark glasses and

the avoidance of bright lights. Intensive psychological counseling, desensitization techniques, and behavioral management should be employed if symptoms progress for more than 4 weeks.

5. Visual scanning and pupillary tracking difficulties may result in significant functional difficulties (eg, reading, driving, work) and should be aggressively investigated (eg, eye gaze testing) and managed (eg, visual rehabilitation).

Vision Deficits

Assessment

While severe vision deficits following polytrauma are relatively uncommon, the potential impact of visual dysfunction on a wide range of functional activities is so significant that all patients should be carefully evaluated to rule them out.

Precautions

A better intervention for diplopia than a patch is the use of translucent tape over one side of a pair of glasses (corrective or cosmetic) or a translucent patch. The translucency prevents the double vision, but also allows light to pass to the eye, which is better tolerated and "normal" feeling.

Management

Partial loss of visual fields (homonymous hemianopsia) is often not noted by the patient. Natural recovery is common by 3 months postinjury, but if recovery is poor, adaptive techniques and orthoptics may be helpful.

Diplopia seems to respond well to eye "patching" on with excellent symptomatic relief for the patient (for both the double vision and the headaches often associated with it).

Visual scanning and pupillary tracking difficulties may result in significant functional difficulties (eg, reading, driving, work) and should be aggressively investigated (eg, eye gaze testing) and managed (eg, visual rehabilitation).

13

Hearing Deficits

1. It's unclear if there are specific hearing deficits directly related to brain injury, although they are common with polytrauma due to the frequency of tympanic membrane ruptures, inner ear damage, and temporal bone fractures. The potential impact of these deficits on a wide range of functional activities is so significant that all patients should be carefully evaluated to rule them out. The impaired processing of the auditory signals by the brain and the understanding of the meaning of those signals by the cognitively impaired patient has been labeled as a "hearing deficit" or by the term "central auditory processing deficit," or "auditory processing disorders." Differentiating this "condition" from the well-established cognitive deficits of traumatic brain injury (TBI) is not clearly elucidated. Oftentimes the patients with the highest chance of having these auditory deficits are those with the most severe brain dysfunction, which limits accurate evaluation as well as the implementation of some of the adaptive and therapeutic strategies available. Individuals

with mild TBI may occasionally have oversensitivity to noise (hyperacusis) and the perception of sound in the absence of corresponding external sound or a phantom sound (tinnitus).

2. Hearing acuity is typically not affected by brain injury, unless it is related to the trauma to the temporal bone, ossicles, or tympanic membrane. Patients who have severe TBI or those with polytrauma who have been exposed to blast injury have a significantly higher likelihood of having sustained an eardrum injury (conductive hearing loss), as well as sensorineural hearing loss. Additionally, individuals with skull fractures of the temporal bone may get an injury to the ear canal, middle ear, inner ear, and vestibulocochlear nerve (cranial nerve VIII) that can result in alterations in hearing acuity, as well as tinnitus, hyperacusis, and balance dysfunction.

3. The most common cause of tinnitus is noise-induced hearing loss, whether from blast injury, munitions discharge, or over-use of earphones, in which sound enters directly into the ear canal without any opportunity to be deflected or absorbed elsewhere. Other causes that should be considered are ototoxic medications, repeated ear infections, foreign objects in the ear, nasal allergies that prevent (or induce) fluid drain, and ear wax buildup. As noted, tinnitus may be an accompaniment of sensorineural hearing loss. As tinnitus is usually a subjective phenomenon, it is difficult to measure using objective tests, such as by comparison with noise of known frequency and intensity, as in an audiometric test. The condition is often rated clinically on a simple scale from "slight" to "catastrophic" according to the practical difficulties it imposes, such as interference with sleep, quiet activities, and normal daily activities. Treatment is focused on

correcting or preventing underlying causes, the use of tinnitus maskers, (noise generators), as well as diet modification (salt restriction, etc.), and stress management.

4. Hyperacusis is often accompanied by tinnitus. It can be viewed as a type of dysesthetic pain, which can quickly develop into a psychological condition (with concomitant pain behaviors). As with all painful conditions, it should be treated acutely (first 2–4 weeks) with "pain blocking agents" that are progressively weaned away as the patient is returned to full activity. In the case of hyperacusis, the blocking agents are not scheduled pain medication, but ear plugs and the avoidance of loud or annoying sounds. Intensive psychological counseling, desensitization techniques, and behavioral management should be employed if symptoms progress for more than 4 weeks.

Hearing Deficits

Assessment

Individuals with mild traumatic brain injury (TBI) may have oversensitivity to noise (hyperacusis). It is sometimes accompanied by the perception of sound in the absence of corresponding external sound or a phantom sound (tinnitus).

Patients with polytrauma who have been exposed to blast injury have a significantly higher likelihood of having sustained an eardrum injury and a sloping high frequency sensorineural hearing loss.

Precautions

The impaired processing of the auditory signals by the brain and the understanding of the meaning of those signals in patients with brain injury have been labeled as "central auditory processing deficit" or "auditory processing disorders."

Differentiating the above condition from the well-established cognitive deficits of TBI requires more research.

Management

Hyperacusis should be treated for the first 2–4 weeks with "pain blocking agents" (ear plugs and the avoidance of loud or annoying sounds) that are progressively weaned away as the patient is returned to full activity.

Intensive psychological counseling, desensitization techniques, and behavioral management should be employed if symptoms progress for more than 4 weeks.

Tinnitus treatment is focused on correcting or preventing underlying causes, the use of tinnitus maskers (noise generators), psychological strategies, diet modification, and stress management.

14

Cranial Nerve Deficits

1. Cranial nerve (CN) injury is not a common result of polytrauma injury. While direct facial trauma may result in peripheral facial (VII) or trigeminal (V) nerve injury, these injuries are rare, rarely functionally impairing, and usually have good outcomes. Severe TBI with either brainstem injury or prolonged elevated intracranial pressures are often accompanied by multiple cranial nerve deficits, including those affecting eye movements (IV, VI), facial movement and sensation (V, VII), hearing (VIII), and swallowing (IX, XII). The most common cranial nerve injury from polytrauma, including concussion, is the olfactory (CN I) nerve, although it often goes undetected and rarely negatively impacts outcome.

2. Brainstem injuries from polytrauma can produce profoundly impairing cranial nerve deficits, oftentimes affecting multiple nerves owing to their close proximity. The functional (speech, vision, swallowing) and cosmetic (facial droop, drooling) difficulties that result can be quite debilitating to the individual and rehabilitation efforts are

largely supportive/adaptive, although these disabilities rarely prevent a return home. Fortunately, most of these patients will gradually recover in the first 3 months postinjury. Little recovery can be expected after 6 months.

3. Deficits in smell (hyposmia, anosmia) are common following TBI, especially when there is frontal cortex damage (ie, the most common site of injury). Unfortunately, unless there is total loss of smell (anosmia), these deficits are often overlooked by clinicians. Individuals are also often unaware unless specifically tested (using standardized smell tests); however, they may manifest it with a decrease in appetite (food taste is 40%–60% associated with smell), an excess use of cologne or perfume, and a failure to note bad food or bodily odors. Treatment is limited to enhancing a patient's awareness of the deficit, recommending food seasonings that stimulate taste buds, and providing adaptive devices for safety (eg, carbon monoxide monitor at home).

Cranial Nerves

Assessment

Brainstem injuries from polytrauma can produce profoundly impairing cranial nerve deficits, oftentimes affecting multiple nerves owing to their close proximity.

The functional and cosmetic difficulties that result can be quite debilitating to the individual. Rehabilitation efforts are largely supportive and adaptive, and they can typically be provided as an outpatient if the individual is otherwise ready to return home.

Precautions

Individuals with olfactory (CN I) nerve deficits will demonstrate decreased appetite and may be at risk to neglect smoke or gas leaks at home.

Management

The most common cranial nerve injury from polytrauma, including concussion, is to the olfactory nerve.

Treatment is limited to enhancing a patient's awareness of the deficit, recommending food seasonings that stimulate taste buds, and providing adaptive devices for safety.

Brainstem injuries are managed with medical optimization, adaptive strategies for deficits (dysphagia, dysarthria, drooling, incomplete eyelid closing), and watchful waiting.

15

Aphasia

1. Aphasia is an acquired impairment of the ability to comprehend and produce language due to brain damage. It is classically associated with ischemic stroke in the middle cerebral artery (MCA) distribution of the language-dominant hemisphere (left hemisphere in over 90% of adults), but can also be seen with traumatic brain injury (TBI) (usually severe) affecting this distribution. It must be differentiated from other impairments that interfere with the ability to follow commands and speak fluently such as hearing impairment, central auditory processing disorders, apraxia of speech, dysarthria, dysfluency, mutism, and executive function deficits.

2. Following polytrauma, individuals with mild to moderate TBI may exhibit evidence of "confused language" that is associated more with their cognitive deficits than true language deficits. Language may demonstrate poor sentence structure, be tangential and echolalic. While these deficits are typically short-lived and directly tied to

improvements in orientation and executive functioning, the elements of impairment fit the definition of aphasia.

3. The cardinal signs of aphasia are impaired comprehension, word-finding deficits (anomia), and paraphasias (incorrect substitution of words or sounds). The impairments of auditory comprehension and speech production are often, but not necessarily and not symmetrically, mirrored by deficits of reading and writing. Patients with a history of CNS insult and evidence of language impairment on bedside neurological exam should be referred to speech-language pathology for thorough aphasia examination. Aphasia is diagnosed, and traditionally classified, via bedside assessment of auditory comprehension (following commands), object naming, repetition of words and phrases, and fluency of conversational speech.

4. The classic aphasia subtypes—Wernicke's, Broca's, conduction, transcortical motor, and transcortical sensory—rarely present in pure form. Within the polytrauma rehabilitation setting, classification of aphasia type is less important than identifying strengths and weaknesses for the purposes of therapeutic intervention.

5. Aphasia therapy involves stimulation of spontaneous recovery of language function as well as teaching compensatory strategies to circumvent current deficits. For patients with severe language comprehension impairments, therapy will be directed toward comprehension of words, phrases, and sentences. Utilization of written materials can be an effective compensatory strategy for patients with better reading ability than auditory comprehension. Picture boards and other augmentative communication devices can facilitate the patient's ability to convey basic wants and needs. For patients with

significant expressive language impairments, therapy will focus on volitional production of functionally relevant words and short phrases. These patients often have significant language comprehension deficits, which are masked by their skill in interpreting facial expression and nonverbal cues that may need to be addressed in therapy. Compensatory strategies may include use of preserved abilities to write and draw as well as augmentative communication devices to circumvent speech production difficulty. Melodic intonation therapy is presumed to recruit intact musical abilities to foster speech production.

6. Aphasia improves with time, but research has shown that in the case of stroke patients, most improvement occurs during the first 3 months, and it is crucial to concentrate therapy during this initial period of spontaneous recovery.

Aphasia

Assessment

Aphasia is diagnosed via bedside assessment of auditory comprehension (following commands), object naming, repetition of words and phrases, and fluency of conversational speech.

Precautions

True aphasia is unusual after polytrauma without focal left frontotemporal lesion.

Confused language is typical of TBI.

Management

Stimulation of spontaneous recovery of language function.

Teaching compensatory strategies to circumvent current deficits.

Utilization of written materials can be an effective compensatory strategy for patients with better reading ability than auditory comprehension. Picture boards and other augmentative communication devices can facilitate the patient's ability to convey basic wants and needs.

Compensatory strategies may include use of preserved abilities to write and draw as well as augmentative communication devices to circumvent speech production difficulty.

Melodic intonation therapy is presumed to recruit intact musical abilities to foster speech production.

Continue to work with speech-language pathology and audiology service during the recovery phase.

Executive Function
Deficits

1. The hallmark of cognitive deficits following traumatic brain injury (TBI) of any severity is abnormalities of executive functioning. Executive functioning is an over-arching term used to describe tasks and abilities that regulate, control, and manage other cognitive processes that originate in the prefrontal areas of the frontal lobe. These functions include planning, working memory, attention, problem solving, verbal reasoning, inhibition, mental flexibility, task switching, initiation, and monitoring of actions. These deficits are the hallmark of mild TBI or concussion, and after any severity of injury executive functioning is the last component of cognition to improve. Permanent deficits of executive functioning are common sequelae of TBI, particularly with more severe or repeated injury.

2. Neuropsychological testing provides the most accurate and valid means of assessing and monitoring executive

functioning. Cognitive therapies to both improve and allow for adaptation (eg, using a daily schedule, setting Smartphone reminders for appointments or for pill taking) for executive functioning deficits are best provided by experienced rehabilitation therapists (psychology, speech and language pathologists, occupational therapists) who adjust their interventions based on both repeated cognitive testing and functional abilities.

3. Medications to enhance executive function recovery have not been research supported; however, they continue to be utilized. After anything that may be sedating or cognitively impairing the patient (eg, alcohol use, centrally acting medications, poor sleep hygiene, lack of physical or cognitive stimulation, systemic infection, hydrocephalus, depression) has been removed, a trial of a medication to enhance arousal (eg, methylphenidate 5–20 mg 2 times daily) may be considered. While stimulating antidepressants (selective serotoninergic reuptake inhibitors [SSRIs]) and other agents (amantadine 100–200 mg 2 times daily) may be considered, their efficacy is unclear and potential side effects must be considered.

Executive Function Deficits

Assessment

Executive functioning is an overarching term to describe tasks and abilities that regulate, control, and manage other cognitive processes and originate in the prefrontal areas of the frontal lobe.

These functions include planning, working memory, attention, problem solving, verbal reasoning, inhibition, mental flexibility, task switching, initiation, and monitoring of actions.

Neuropsychological testing provides the most accurate and valid means of assessing and monitoring executive functioning.

Precautions

While stimulating antidepressants (SSRIs) and other agents (amantadine) may be considered, their efficacy is unclear and potential side effects must be considered.

Management

All potentially sedating or cognitively impairing agents or conditions must be addressed.

Cognitive therapies to both improve and allow for adaptation (eg, using a daily schedule, setting Smartphone reminders for appointments or for pill taking) for executive functioning deficits are best provided by experienced rehabilitation therapists (psychology, speech and language pathologists, occupational therapists) who adjust their interventions based on both repeated cognitive testing and functional abilities.

Medications to enhance executive function recovery have not been research supported; however, they continue to be utilized. Methylphenidate is the most widely used and accepted.

Akinetic Mutism and Locked-In Syndrome

1. Akinetic mutism is a condition, often confused with a disorder of consciousness (coma), in which patients have limited movement (akinesia) and speech (mutism) as a result of severe frontal lobe injury. It is also known as abulia and has been associated with psychologic and psychogenic conditions. The deficits are felt to be due to difficulty with motor initiation from frontal lobe damage.

2. Locked-in syndrome (LIS) must be considered in individuals with akinetic mutism. In LIS, individuals have awareness, sleep-wake cycles, and meaningful behavior (eg, eye movement), but have no movement due to quadriplegia and pseudobulbar palsy. Thus, these patients are aware and awake but cannot move or communicate verbally due to complete paralysis of nearly all voluntary muscles in the body; however, often the

eyes/eye blinks can still have purposeful movement. Total LIS is a version of LIS where the eyes are paralyzed as well. Patients with LIS have no movement, including speech, related to a pontine injury/insult that essentially isolates the cerebral cortex from the cranial and motor nerves. Unlike akinetic mutism, the deficits are unrelated to initiation and these patients will have intact cognition (unless a cortical injury is also present) and can typically use their eyes/eye blinks to communicate.

3. Once it has been confirmed that the individual is neither comatose nor has a medical condition (subclinical seizures, hydrocephalus, LIS) preventing motor/speech initiation, efforts are directed at facilitating activity (eg, putting an individual in an automatic activity such as singing basic songs, catching a ball, or clapping). While natural recovery will usually allow for improvements, for patients who continue to have limitations, medication intervention (eg, methylphenidate, bromocriptine) may be considered.

Akinetic Mutism

Assessment

Assess patient's communication and motor abilities using standard techniques.

Precautions

Rule out disorder of consciousness (coma, vegetative state, etc.).

Rule out locked-in syndrome.

Rule out seizures and hydrocephalus.

Management

Attempt to elicit automatic movements or speech.

Provide structured rehabilitation therapies focused on repeated activities and speech.

Poor prognosis if persists past 3 months.

18

Posttraumatic Amnesia

1. Posttraumatic amnesia (PTA) is a deficit in memory caused by trauma with brain injury. The memory can be either completely or partially lost due to the extent of damage. There are two main types of amnesia: retrograde amnesia and anterograde amnesia. Retrograde amnesia is the inability to retrieve information that was acquired before a particular date, usually the date of an accident or operation. In some cases the memory loss can extend back decades, while in others the person may lose only a few months of memory. Anterograde amnesia is the inability to transfer new information from the short-term store into the long-term store. People with this type of amnesia cannot remember things for long periods of time. These two types are not mutually exclusive. Both can occur within a patient at one time.

2. The duration of anterograde PTA after traumatic brain injury (TBI) is directly related to the severity of injury (eg, a mild TBI can be defined by a PTA <1 hour, moderate TBI can be defined by PTA <1 day) and is also a moderately

useful prognosticator of long-term outcome. It is unclear whether retrograde amnesia has similar associations.

3. Emergence from anterograde PTA is determined when the patient is able to form new memories, most often measured by orientation to place, time, and situation. Scientifically, PTA is monitored using the Galveston Orientation and Amnesia Test (GOAT) and emergence from PTA is marked by a score of 75 or more on the GOAT for 3 consecutive days (PTA emergence is then determined to be the first such day).

4. As with all cognitive deficits after TBI, amnesia is managed by a variety of measures, including medical management, sleep hygiene, environmental structure, daily schedules, repeated reorientation and memory training, and a return to premorbid (over learned) activities.

Amnesia

Assessment

Utilize Galveston Orientation and Amnesia test (GOAT).

Amnesia has resolved when GOAT is ≥ 75 for 3 consecutive days.

Agitation present if ABS ≥ 21.

Precautions

Duration of posttraumatic amnesia (PTA) correlates with outcome.

Acute infection, seizures, and effects of sedative medications can mimic amnesia.

Management

Medical management

Sleep hygiene

Environmental structure

Daily schedules

Repeated reorientation and memory training

Return to premorbid (over learned) activities

19

Perceptual Deficits

1. Injury to the right parietal lobe (as well as linkages between the parietal, temporal, and occipital lobes) can result in disorders of perception, most commonly visual. The deficits can range from mild visual field cuts to inability to recognize objects (agnosia) to complete inattention or neglect (hemiagnosia) to one side (typically the left). Right-sided spatial neglect is rare because there is redundant processing of the right space by both the left and right cerebral hemispheres, whereas in most left-dominant brains the left space is only processed by the right cerebral hemisphere. Additionally, the right hemisphere of the brain is specialized for spatial perception and memory, whereas the left hemisphere is specialized for language—there is redundant processing of the right visual fields by both hemispheres. Although it most strikingly affects visual perception, neglect in other forms of perception can also be found, either alone or in combination with visual neglect.

2. Agnosia, spatial perception deficits, and neglect are from visual deficits, such as hemianopsia (loss of vision in half the visual field of each eye). Hemianopsia arises from damage to the primary visual pathways cutting off the input to the cerebral hemispheres from the retinas. Visual perceptual deficits are due to damage to the processing areas. The cerebral hemispheres receive the input, but there is an error in the processing that is not well understood. Perceptual deficits not only affect present sensation but memory and recall perception as well. A patient suffering from neglect, for example, may also, when asked to recall a memory of a certain object and then draw said object again, only draw half of the object. It is unclear, however, if this is due to a perceptive deficit of the memory (having lost pieces of spatial information of the memory) or whether the information within the memory is whole and intact, but simply being ignored, the same way portions of a physical object in the patient's presence would be ignored.

3. The lack of attention to the left side of space can manifest in the visual, auditory, proprioceptive, and olfactory domains. Although hemispatial perceptual deficits often manifest as a sensory deficit (and are frequently comorbid with sensory deficit), they are essentially a failure to pay sufficient attention to sensory input. This is particularly evident in a related, but separate, condition known as extinction. A patient with extinction following right-hemisphere damage will successfully report the presence of an object in left space when it is the only object present. However, if the same object is presented simultaneously with an object in right space, the patient will only report the object on the right.

4. Examination of visual-spatial ability is accomplished by asking the patient to draw simple figures, such as a flower, square, or the face of a clock. Completing pencil-and-paper mazes also reveals visual spatial ability. Block puzzle tasks are also used to examine the patient's ability to form 2- and 3-dimensional constructions. Usually the patient is asked to reproduce a block shape shown in a picture or assembled by the examiner. Errors in routefinding and topographical orientation are assessed by self-report of the patient or by an interview of the patient's spouse or family. They will usually have a few stories about the patient's difficulties that clearly suggest the patient gets lost or cannot coordinate the body in space.

5. Treatments to improve perceptual deficits are of unclear efficacy; however, fortunately some degree of spontaneous recovery is common. Intervention efforts focus on identifying and reminding the deficit to patients, providing compensatory strategies (eg, highlighting the left side of objects with bright colors, teaching patients to over scan to the left), and utilizing acoustic (eg, bells), tactile (eg, weights, pressure wraps), and visual (eg, lights, bright colors) cueing on the left limbs and providing excess stimuli (eg, low level electrical) to the affected side or trunk (usually neck) to attempt to "reteach" the brain. Medication interventions do not appear to have any meaningful role.

Perceptual Deficits

Assessment

Examination of visual-spatial ability is accomplished by asking the patient to draw simple figures, such as a flower, square, or the face of a clock.

Completing pencil-and-paper mazes also reveals visual spatial ability.

Block puzzle tasks are also used to examine the patient's ability to form 2- and 3-dimensional constructions.

Usually the patient is asked to reproduce a block shape shown in a picture or assembled by the examiner.

Precautions

Errors in routefinding and topographical orientation are assessed by self-report of the patient, assessment of the patient's drawing and maze testing, or by an interview of the patient's spouse or family.

Management

Treatments to improve perceptual deficits are of unclear efficacy; however, fortunately some degree of spontaneous recovery is common.

Intervention efforts focus on identifying and reminding the deficit to patients, providing compensatory strategies (eg, highlighting the left side of objects with bright colors, teaching patients to over scan to the left), and utilizing acoustic (eg, bells), tactile (eg, weights, pressure wraps), and visual (eg, lights, bright colors) cueing on the left limbs and providing excess stimuli (eg, low level electrical) to the affected side or trunk (usually neck) to attempt to "reteach" the brain.

Medication interventions do not appear to have any meaningful role.

Neglect

1. Unilateral inattention or neglect (hemiagnosia) occurs when damage to one hemisphere of the brain is sustained, and a deficit in attention to and awareness of one side (typically the opposite side as the brain damage) of space is observed. Neglect is most closely related to damage to the temporoparietal junction and posterior parietal cortex. It is defined by the inability of a person to process and perceive stimuli on one side of the body or environment that is not due to a lack of sensation. Neglect results most commonly from brain injury to the right cerebral hemisphere, causing visual neglect of the left-hand side of space. Right-sided spatial neglect is rare because there is redundant processing of the right space by both the left and right cerebral hemispheres, whereas in most left-dominant brains, the left space is only processed by the right cerebral hemisphere. Additionally, the right hemisphere of the brain is specialized for spatial perception and memory, whereas the left hemisphere is specialized for language—there is redundant processing

of the right visual fields by both hemispheres. Although it most strikingly affects visual perception, neglect in other forms of perception can also be found, either alone, or in combination with visual neglect.

2. Neglect is not to be confused with hemianopsia (visual deficits in half the visual field of each eye). Hemianopsia arises from damage to the primary visual pathways cutting off the input to the cerebral hemispheres from the retinas. Neglect is damage to the processing areas. The cerebral hemispheres receive the input, but there is an error in the processing that is not well understood. Neglect not only affects present sensation but memory and recall perception as well. A patient suffering from neglect may also, when asked to recall a memory of a certain object and then draw said object again, only draw half of the object. It is unclear, however, if this is due to a perceptive deficit of the memory (having lost pieces of spatial information of the memory) or whether the information within the memory is whole and intact, but simply being ignored, the same way portions of a physical object in the patient's presence would be ignored.

3. The lack of attention to the left side of space can manifest in the visual, auditory, proprioceptive, and olfactory domains. Although hemispatial neglect often manifests as a sensory deficit (and is frequently comorbid with sensory deficit), it is essentially a failure to pay sufficient attention to sensory input. This is particularly evident in a related, but separate, condition known as extinction. A patient with extinction following right-hemisphere damage will successfully report the presence of an object in left space when it is the only object present.

However, if the same object is presented simultaneously with an object in right space, the patient will only report the object on the right.

4. While treatments to improve neglect are of unclear efficacy, fortunately some degree of spontaneous recovery is common. Intervention efforts focus on identifying and reminding the deficit to patients, providing compensatory strategies (eg, highlighting the left side of objects with bright colors, teaching patients to over scan to the left), and utilizing acoustic (eg, bells), tactile (eg, weights, pressure wraps) and visual (eg, lights, bright colors) cueing on the left limbs and providing excess stimuli (eg, low level electrical) to the affected side or trunk (usually neck) to attempt to "reteach" the brain. Medication interventions do not appear to have any meaningful role.

Neglect

Assessment

Neglect not only affects present sensation but memory and recall perception as well.

When asked to recall a certain object from memory and then draw said object again, a patient suffering from neglect may draw only half of the object.

Precautions

Right-sided spatial neglect is rare because there is redundant processing of the right space by both the left and right cerebral hemispheres, whereas in most left-dominant brains, the left space is only processed by the right cerebral hemisphere.

Management

While treatments to improve neglect are of unclear efficacy, fortunately some degree of spontaneous recovery is common.

Intervention efforts focus on identifying and reminding the deficit to patients, providing compensatory strategies (eg, highlighting the left side of objects with bright colors, teaching patients to over scan to the left), and utilizing acoustic (eg, bells), tactile (eg, weights, pressure wraps) and visual (eg, lights, bright colors) cueing on the left limbs and providing excess stimuli (eg, low level electrical) to the affected side or trunk (usually neck) to attempt to "reteach" the brain.

Medication interventions do not appear to have any meaningful role.

21

Agitation, Irritability, and Emotional Lability

1. Agitation is expected after moderate to severe traumatic brain injury (TBI) and may actually be a sign of progress during recovery from a disorder of consciousness (DOC). Careful evaluation of the time course, underlying cause(s) of agitation, and response to nonpharmacologic interventions are vital to the appropriate management of and the avoidance of complications associated with agitation (and its treatment) that may impede rehabilitation. Agitation may be defined as a subtype of delirium occurring in the state of posttraumatic amnesia, characterized by excesses of behavior, including some combination of aggression, akathisia, disinhibition, and/or emotional lability.

2. A crucial step in the management of agitation is objective measurement of its characterization and severity. Two commonly used instruments are the Agitated Behavior Scale (ABS) and the Overt Agitation Severity Scale (OASS).

Behaviors captured as agitation may usually be grouped into aggression, disinhibition, or emotional.

3. The ABS quantifies 14 unique behaviors observed over a specified period (usually 8–12 hours) and rates them as absent (1), present to a slight degree (2), present to a moderate degree (3), or present to an extreme degree (4). A total score of 21 or below is considered normal, while scores of 22 to 28, 29 to 35, and 35 to 56 are classified as mild, moderate, and severe agitation, respectively.

4. The OASS rates the severity of 47 distinct behaviors, taking into account their frequency of occurrence.

5. Management of agitation requires direct observation of the patient in the environment in which the agitation is occurring. Modification of the environment to eliminate factors that contribute to or precipitate agitation should be the initial step of management and should be common practice for all individuals with TBI. A frequent cause of agitation is excessive environmental stimulation, thus, for example, unnecessary noise such as TVs and radios should be turned off. Limiting the number of visitors and/or moderating their behavior may be a key step.

6. Therapists and nurses may contribute to agitation if they say too much or speak at the same time as others. They should talk to the patient in a normal tone of voice and use short, direct utterances, communicating one idea at a time. Consistency in terms of nursing care will reduce confusion.

7. If at all possible, stimuli such as catheters, IV lines, and restraints should be discontinued. Restraints should be minimal and should only be employed if the patient is a danger to himself or herself or others. Use of restraints requires careful supervision to prevent self-injury.

8. When possible, patient restlessness should be permitted and accommodated into therapy and nursing care, often with assistance of the family. Simple floor beds, veiled beds, wall padding, and one-to-one supervision may allow the patient to thrash about in bed and/or move around the unit safely.

9. Medical causes of agitation must be investigated prior to initiation of pharmacologic treatment. Such causes include infection, fracture, seizure, hydrocephalus, intracranial hemorrhage, dyspnea, musculoskeletal pain, pressure ulcers, urinary retention or incontinence, constipation, medication side effects, overdose or withdrawal, withdrawal from illicit substances, electrolyte derangement, hepatic encephalopathy, and endocrine disorder.

10. Agitation of at least moderate severity that persists despite environmental modification and investigation of medical etiologies may be managed with medication. The classes of medications available include antipsychotics, beta blockers, anticonvulsants, antidepressants, and benzodiazepines. The lowest therapeutic dosing that improves the agitation (ie, reduces ABS/OASS scores to nonagitated) should be used. Once agitation has improved, a rapid taper over 3–5 days is usually feasible without relapse.

11. The most commonly used typical antipsychotics are haloperidol and chlorpromazine. They have been shown to retard recovery in TBI patients and are typically used for short-term management until other agents can be adequately titrated or for patients who are poorly responsive to other traditional agents. Atypical antipsychotics may be preferable to typical antipsychotics due to fewer side effects and decreased risk of movement disorders. Members of this class include risperidone, ziprasidone, quetiapine, and aripiprazole.

12. Beta blockers, such as propranolol, have been shown efficacious for agitation associated with aggression (rage or violent behavior) and usually do not have significant cardiovascular limitations from hypotension and bradycardia. Dosing should begin at 10 to 20 mg 3 times daily and then titrated up daily to 60 mg total dosing daily until agitation is manageable, taking into account cardiovascular parameters.

13. Anticonvulsants, such as valproic acid, lamotrigine, and carbamazepine, are good options for persistent disinhibition (restlessness or impulsivity), but may impede cognitive recovery. Dosing should be titrated up rapidly using standard anticonvulsant serum levels as maximal dosing indicators.

14. Tricyclic antidepressants are used less commonly, but may have a therapeutic effect on agitation with features of emotional lability. Nortriptyline is the preferred agent and serum levels for depression usage may be used as maximal dosing indicators. Study results have been mixed on the use of antidepressants such as sertraline, amitriptyline, buspirone, and fluvoxamine.

15. Benzodiazepines such as lorazepam and midazolam should be used sparingly due to their negative effect upon recovery. Of note, this class of medications may cause paradoxical agitation in some patients.

16. Physicians using antipsychotics and antidepressants for agitation management should be on alert for side effects and potentially devastating complications such as neuroleptic malignant syndrome. Typical signs and symptoms of neuroleptic malignant syndrome include fever, stiffness, leukocytosis, rhabdomyolysis, and kidney failure. It can be managed with beta blockers and dantrolene.

Agitation, Irritability, and Emotional Lability

Assessment

Utilize Agitated Behavior Scale (ABS)

Monitor ABS q8–12 for 72 hours

Agitation present if ABS ≥ 21

Precautions

Rule out drivers of agitation (pain, infection, hypoxia, drugs, alcohol)

Rule out seizures and hydrocephalus

Management

ABS < 28

Reduce environmental distractions

Establish a steady routine

Normalize sleep

As needed Ativan or Risperidone (1 mg PO/IM) every 4 hours overnight

ABS = 28–56

For aggression, start propranolol at 10–20 mg tid and increase by 60 mg daily

For restlessness, start carbamazepine 100 mg tid and titrate to serum level

For emotional lability, start nortriptyline 25 mg qhs and increase by 25 mg daily to 150 mg total

Depression

1. Depression is the most common major mental illness that has been associated with traumatic brain injury (TBI), with some research noting an incidence as high as 50% in the first year after injury. While some literature supports an elevated incidence of posttraumatic depression in individuals with left frontal injury or insult, clinicians should maintain an awareness of it in all patients. Similarly, while more severe injuries seem to have elevated incidences of associated depression, all injury severities have a significantly elevated risk for at least the first year postinjury. Individuals with the severest injuries will continue to have a clinically relevant increased risk for 3 or more years postinjury.

2. Sadness, a depressed affect, or intermittent periods of "feeling blue" or down (dysthymia) are common in all individuals and most likely occurs more often in those with acute physical limitations. These transient alterations in mood are normal reactions to life, pain, insomnia, and alterations in daily activities. Interventions

should be directed at improving these vegetative signs and difficulties, with specific emphasis on exercise, nutrition, relaxation training, adjustment counseling, pain management, and sleep hygiene. There is no role for antidepressant medications in these individuals, as they do not have depression ("major depression").

3. Depression or major depressive disorder (MDD) is typified by a very low mood, which pervades all aspects of life, and an inability to experience pleasure in activities that were formerly enjoyed. Depressed people may be preoccupied with, or ruminate over, thoughts and feelings of worthlessness, inappropriate guilt or regret, helplessness, hopelessness, and self-hatred. In severe cases, depressed people may have symptoms of psychosis. These symptoms include delusions or, less commonly, hallucinations, usually unpleasant. Other symptoms of depression include poor concentration and memory (especially in those with melancholic or psychotic features), withdrawal from social situations and activities, reduced sex drive, and thoughts of death or suicide. Insomnia is common among the depressed.

4. The Structural Clinical Interview for *DSM-IV* (SCID), a clinical interview that uses the *DSM-IV* criteria for illness, is the gold standard for the (research) diagnosis of depression, however depression must be diagnosed through a detailed history, exam, and testing (to rule out TBI or physiologic causes of vegetative signs and symptoms). Commonly used self-report measures to assist clinicians are the Center for Epidemiological Study of Depression Scale (CES-D), and the Beck Depression Inventory (BDI). Frequent assessment of the individual's risk for suicidality must always be monitored, given the significant association between depression and suicide.

Making the diagnosis of depression in individuals with TBI can be challenging because of both the overlap of signs and symptoms commonly seen in the two conditions and the challenge of interviewing and examining individuals with significant cognitive and motoric deficits.

5. Treatment of MDD after TBI must be multimodal and take into considerations the cognitive, behavioral and physical limitations that are present from the TBI. Nutrition, exercise, pain conditions, and insomnia should be optimized. Psychological therapy, specifically cognitive behavioral therapy, is the gold standard of care and has been demonstrated to be equally effective in individuals with TBI (program modifications for cognitive deficits should be made). Oftentimes antidepressants are used concomitantly, although the efficacy is only fair. Of note, antidepressants (eg, selective serotonine reuptake inhibitors) must be adequately dosed and those dosages adjusted based on effects and side effects. Given the self-report nature of symptom monitoring, the cognitive/memory abilities of the individual must be accounted for and adaptive strategies utilized (eg, relying on family members, using a log book or Smartphone app). Short-term usage of antidepressants (ie, less than 1 year) have been associated with an elevated risk of relapse, so a long-term commitment is required by both the patient and clinician.

Depression

Assessment

The Structural Clinical Interview for *DSM-IV* (SCID), a clinical interview that uses the *DSM-IV* criteria for mental and personality disorders, is the gold standard for the (research) diagnosis of depression.

Depression must be diagnosed through a detailed history, exam, and testing.

Commonly used self-report measures to assist clinicians are the Center for Epidemiological Study of Depression Scale (CES-D), and the Beck Depression Inventory (BDI).

Precautions

Frequent assessment of the individual's risk for suicidality must always be monitored, given the significant association between depression and suicide.

Management

Treatment must be multimodal and take into consideration the cognitive, behavioral, and physical limitations that are present from the traumatic brain injury (TBI).

Nutrition, exercise, pain conditions, and insomnia should be optimized.

Psychological therapy, specifically cognitive behavioral therapy, is the gold standard of care and has been demonstrated to be equally effective in individuals with TBI.

Antidepressants are often used but the efficacy is only fair. Short-term usage of antidepressants (ie, less than 1 year) have been associated with an elevated risk of relapse, so a long-term commitment is required by both the patient and clinician.

Hypoarousal

1. Following polytrauma with moderate to severe traumatic brain injury (TBI), particularly with subcortical injury, difficulties in maintaining arousal are common. Regulation of arousal (and sleep-wake transitions) is controlled by the reticular activating system (RAS), or extrathalamic control modulatory system, which is a set of connected nuclei in the brain that link in the brainstem through the reticular formation. The reticular formation filters incoming stimuli to discriminate irrelevant background stimuli. Thus, in addition to poor arousal (hypoarousal), individuals with injury to these pathways also have difficulty with attentional tasks. Hypoarousal is a prognosticator for poor functional recovery.

2. In addition to optimizing care (eg, monitoring for hydrocephalus, seizures, infection, hypoxia, metabolic, and endocrinologic abnormalities) to allow for natural recovery after injury, rehabilitative interventions to facilitate improvement of arousal (and attention) include normalizing sleep-wake cycles through appropriate sleep

hygiene, eliminating distracting background environment stimulation (eg, television, cluttered rooms, excess light), establishing a schedule with periods of focused and appropriate stimuli (eg, nondistracting environment, specific tasking, no sedating medications) alternating with controlled periods of rest, and eliminating medications that may be sedating or confusing.

3. Often medications that provide activation may be beneficial (although rarely curative), including certain antidepressants (especially if concomitant depression is suspected), amantadine, and methylphenidate. Methylphenidate has the most rapid and specific effect and should be considered as a first-line agent (5–20 mg given in the morning and at lunch). Once sufficient arousal (and attention) have been achieved to allow for participation and gains in functional activities, these medication should be weaned.

Hypoarousal

Assessment

Arousal can be best assessed by determining the degree of attention available to allow for participation and gains in functional activities.

Neuropsychological testing provides the most accurate and valid means of assessing and monitoring attention; however, most patients with hypoarousal state cannot tolerate these lengthy batteries.

Precautions

In addition to poor arousal (hypoarousal), individuals with injury to the reticular activating system pathways will also have difficulty with attentional tasks.

Hypoarousal is a prognosticator for poor functional recovery.

Management

Hypoarousal management includes:

- Optimizing care (eg, monitoring for hydrocephalus, seizures, infection, hypoxia, metabolic and endocrinologic abnormalities) to allow for natural recovery after injury
- Normalizing sleep-wake cycles through appropriate sleep hygiene
- Eliminating distracting background environment stimulation
- Establishing a schedule with periods of focused and appropriate stimuli alternating with controlled periods of rest
- Eliminating medications that may be sedating or confusing

Methylphenidate has the most rapid and specific effect and should be considered as a first-line agent.

Sexual Dysfunction

1. Long-term physical and physiological abnormalities that result in sexual dysfunction are rare after polytrauma, while acute difficulties (eg, pain, mobility, fatigue) are common. This is also true for fertility (male and female). Unfortunately, due to the cognitive and behavioral challenges that result from polytrauma, difficulties with sexuality (the capacity to have erotic experiences and responses) are more common. Clinicians must be aware and comfortable in addressing all aspects of an individual's status (eg, physical, emotional, cultural) and social situation when managing issues related to sex and sexuality.

2. Traumatic brain injury (TBI) issues related to sexual dysfunction tend to be related to cognitive (eg, inability to regulate social interactions, ease of distractibility), behavioral (eg, inappropriate comments, intrusiveness, irritability, hypersexuality), physical (eg, pain, mobility limitation, spasticity, coordination), and endocrinologic (eg, low testosterone, hypothyroidism, lower cortisol levels), function

which can be addressed with traditional rehabilitative interventions. Taking into consideration an individual's cultural and social background is a vital piece of the evaluation and management of both sexual function and sexuality. Similarly, the clinician must consider the degree of recovery and the persistence of deficits in cognition and behavior before addressing sexuality and make adaptations for these deficits, if feasible. True neurologic deficits that directly impact sexual functioning from TBI are extremely rare. On the other hand, most injuries to the spinal cord (or peripheral sacral nerves) will result in neurologic (as well as physical) challenges to sexual function both acutely and chronically. Direct trauma to genitalia (including penile/scrotal amputation) from blast injury polytrauma presents unique challenges, both related to reconstructive surgery (which rarely produces functional results, but may have profoundly positive cosmetic and psychological outcomes) and addressing alternative approaches to sexual function and sexuality.

3. Fortunately, the current medications for erectile dysfunction (eg, sildenafil, tadalafil) are typically effective regardless of neurologic dysfunction. In addition to the medical precautions that must be considered with these agents (ie, cardiovascular), the clinician must also consider the level of cognitive/behavioral abilities, physical abilities (including sensation and skin integrity), and concomitant medical conditions. Other interventions available include penile vacuum devices, the use of adaptive aids, and injected medications. A return to sexual activity is usually physically safe 6 weeks after an intracranial event or procedure; however, all recommendations should be individualized.

4. Male and female fertility following polytrauma is typically negatively affected in the first 1–12 months (depending on the severity of injury and secondary medical issues); however, fertility usually returns to baseline long term. Persistent hormonal and medical abnormalities may delay recovery and should be investigated if infertility persists after 12 months. Importantly, individuals should be counseled early, often, and honestly about safe sexual practices, as fertility usually returns to normal and sexually transmitted diseases remain an issue regardless.

Sexual Dysfunction

Assessment

Clinicians must be aware of and comfortable in addressing all aspects of an individual's status (eg, physical, emotional, cultural) and social situation when managing issues related to sexual function and sexuality in general.

Precautions

Individuals with polytrauma should be counseled early, often, and honestly about safe sexual practices, as fertility usually returns to normal and sexually transmitted diseases remain an issue regardless.

Management

Traumatic brain injury (TBI) issues related to sexual dysfunction tend to be related to cognitive, behavioral, physical, and endocrinologic function, which can be addressed with traditional rehabilitative interventions.

Taking into consideration an individual's cultural and social background is a vital piece of the evaluation and management of both sexual function and sexuality.

Clinician must consider the degree of recovery and the persistence of deficits in cognition and behavior before addressing sexuality, and make adaptations for these deficits, if feasible.

True neurologic deficits that directly impact sexual functioning from TBI are. On the other hand, most injuries to the spinal cord will result in neurologic challenges to sexual function both acutely and chronically.

Direct trauma to genitalia from blast injury polytrauma presents unique challenges, both related to reconstructive surgery and addressing alternative approaches to sexual function and sexuality.

Neurogenic Bladder

1. The physiatrist working in the polytrauma setting should be familiar with the common patterns of bladder dysfunction seen in stroke, traumatic brain injury (TBI), and spinal cord injury (SCI), and their associated management strategies.

2. The three most common types of neurogenic bladder are lower motor neuron (LMN) bladder (flaccid bladder with failure to empty), upper motor neuron (UMN) bladder (hyperactive or spastic bladder with failure to store), and detrusor-sphincter dyssynergia (DSD; combination spastic bladder with inability to empty). In LMN bladder, there is urinary retention and overflow incontinence at high volumes due to flaccidity of the bladder or incompetence of the internal sphincter. Patients with UMN bladder tend to have incontinence due to frequent, low-volume voiding attributable to hyperreflexic bladder contractions and/or spasticity of the internal sphincter. In DSD there is spasm of the detrusor muscle and the

internal sphincter with resulting urinary retention, high intravesical pressure, and risk of vesicoureteral reflux.

3. The diagnosis of neurogenic bladder begins with patient or caregiver history regarding frequency of voiding, episodes of incontinence, and history of urinary tract infections (UTI). Other initial diagnostic steps include measurement of voiding volumes, bladder scans to determine postvoid residuals, and checking for UTI with urinalysis and urine culture. These basic diagnostic steps should allow for rough classification of type of bladder dysfunction and guide implementation of initial management strategies.

4. For patients with LMN bladder due to SCI, cauda equina lesion, or peripheral neuropathy (diabetes mellitus), basic management options include indwelling Foley catheter or/and intermittent catheterization. Condom catheters rarely suffice due to the inability of the bladder to completely empty. Because indwelling catheters increase the risk of UTI, intermittent catheterization is preferred in almost all cases. Patients should be catheterized 4 to 5 times per day, more frequently if volumes exceed 500 mL. With SCI at or above the T6 level, bladder overdistension is the most common trigger for autonomic dysreflexia. Pharmacologic treatment options for LMN bladder include cholinergics, such as bethanecol and alpha blockers such as terazosin. This option is suboptimal due to limited efficacy and bothersome side effects (drooling, sweating, diarrhea).

5. UMN bladder, common in the acute and subacute stages of cerebrovascular accident (stroke) (CVA) or TBI and in cervical or thoracic SCI, is best treated initially with timed voiding to prevent incontinent episodes. Anticholinergics, such as ditropan, antimuscurinics, such as tolteridine, and

tricyclic antidepressants (TCAs), such as nortriptyline, to relax the bladder, are pharmacologic options.

6. DSD, most commonly seen in individuals with cervical and high thoracic SCI, is often more challenging to treat; however, behavioral strategies such as timed voids and intermittent catheterization may be effective. Anticholinergics to relax the bladder and alpha blockers to relax the internal sphincter are reasonable options. Surgical options include ablation of fibers of the external sphincter or bladder neck, placement of a suprapubic catheter, or bladder diversion.

7. A urodynamic study, in which the bladder is filled with fluid and pressures, volumes, and muscle activity are measured throughout the storage and voiding phases of bladder function, allows for thorough assessment of bladder physiology and is commonly recommended initially for all individuals with SCI after they have emerged from "spinal shock." Urodynamics are rarely useful during the acute stage of polytrauma rehabilitation but are essential prior to decision making regarding definitive management of neurogenic bladder.

8. Patients with risk of vesicoureteral reflux should undergo yearly ultrasound of the upper urinary tract for detection of hydronephrosis.

9. Patients with indwelling catheters need cystoscopy every 5 to 10 years for surveillance of bladder cancer.

Neurogenic Bladder

Assessment

The diagnosis of neurogenic bladder begins with patient or caregiver history regarding frequency of voiding, episodes of incontinence, and history of urinary tract infections (UTI).

Other initial diagnostic steps include measurement of voiding volumes, bladder scans to determine postvoid residuals, and checking for UTI with urinalysis and urine culture.

Precautions

Patients with risk of vesicoureteral reflux should undergo yearly ultrasound of the upper urinary tract for detection of hydronephrosis.

With spinal cord injury at or above the T6 level, bladder overdistension is the most common trigger for autonomic dysreflexia.

Management

Basic management options for lower motor neuron (LMN) bladder includes indwelling Foley catheter or intermittent catheterization. For males, condom catheters rarely suffice due to the inability of the bladder to completely empty. Because indwelling catheters increase the risk of UTI, intermittent catheterization is preferred in most cases.

Upper motor neuron (UMN) bladder is best treated initially with timed voiding to prevent incontinent episodes. Anticholinergics, such as ditropan, antimuscurinics, such as tolteridine, and TCAs, such as nortriptyline, to relax the bladder, are pharmacologic options.

26

Neurogenic Bowel

1. The physiatrist working in the polytrauma setting should be familiar with the common patterns of bowel dysfunction seen in stroke, traumatic brain injury (TBI), and spinal cord injury (SCI) and their associated management strategies. Neurogenic bowel dysfunction is common in acute stroke or TBI, and often chronically problematic in SCI, multiple sclerosis, ALS, and neuromuscular disorders. It can be seriously detrimental to quality of life, preventing social and vocational interaction. The two most common types of neurogenic bowel are lower motor neuron (LMN) bladder (flaccid bowel with failure to empty) and upper motor neuron (UMN) bladder (hyperactive or spastic bowel with failure to empty).

2. Patients with LMN bowel, seen in chonus medullaris or cauda equina SCI, have prolonged colonic transit times, especially distally, and resulting constipation, with the further complication of incontinence due to a flaccid external sphincter.

3. UMN bowel is most common in SCI above the level of the conus medullaris and is characterized by prolonged colonic transit times and decreased urge to defecate with resulting constipation, fecal impaction, and, sometimes, liquid incontinence around impacted stool.

4. Neurogenic bowel dysfunction is initially assessed with a thorough history and physical exam. Key aspects of the history include premorbid bowel function, current level of activity, diet, current medications, and current bowel program. During the physical exam, careful assessment of the abdomen and examination of the anus are important. For patients with neuromuscular disease, strength, dexterity, and range of motion of the upper extremities must be assessed to predict the patient's level of independence with bowel care.

5. Plain films of the abdomen are helpful in ruling out impaction and obstruction. Guaiac is often indicated to rule out bleeding. More invasive testing such as endoscopy, manometry/pressure measurement, and electromyogram (EMG) may be considered.

6. The goals of neurogenic bowel management programs are to have regular, planned bowel movements and to avoid incontinence and complications. The neurogenic bowel patient's intake should include 2 to 3 L of water per day and 15 to 30 g of fiber per day.

7. If at all possible, constipating medications such as opioids and anticholinergics should be discontinued in favor of more bowel-friendly alternatives. For UMN bowel, a good initial regimen is a stool softener such as docusate sodium twice daily and an agent that stimulates peristalsis such as senna once daily. If oral agents alone are insufficient, a suppository such as bisacodyl

or glycerine may be necessary. For LMN bowel, a bulk-forming agent such as psyllium or methylcellulose may be effective. Digital stimulation by the patient or caregiver with a gloved and lubricated finger will help to stimulate defecation via the anorectal reflex. For some patients, manual removal of the stool may be necessary.

8. Timing of components of the bowel program to take advantage of gravity and GI reflexes is an important consideration. In order to utilize the gastrocolic reflex, which is colonic contractions triggered by distension of the stomach, the patient should do his or her bowel program about 30 minutes after a meal.

9. Colostomy is a management option for patients who are unable to perform a successful bowel program and may enhance quality of life significantly for patients suffering from complications of neurogenic bowel such as skin breakdown, urinary tract infections, and obstruction secondary to fecal impaction.

Neurogenic Bowel

Assessment

Neurogenic bowel dysfunction is initially assessed with a thorough history and physical exam.

Key aspects of the history include premorbid bowel function, current level of activity, diet, current medications, and current bowel program.

During the physical exam, careful assessment of the abdomen and examination of the anus are important. For patients with neuromuscular disease, strength, dexterity, and range of motion of the upper extremities must be assessed to predict the patient's level of independence with bowel care.

Precautions

Neurogenic bowel dysfunction is common in polytrauma, acute stroke or TBI, and is often chronically problematic in SCI, multiple sclerosis, ALS, and neuromuscular disorders.

It can be seriously detrimental to quality of life, preventing social and vocational interaction.

Management

The goals of neurogenic bowel management programs are to have regular, planned bowel movements and to avoid incontinence and complications.

A patient with neurogenic bowel should have an intake of at least 2–3 L of water per day and 15–30 g of fiber per day.

Postconcussive Syndrome

1. Physical, cognitive, and behavioral symptoms commonly occur acutely (ie, within the first 2 weeks) after mild traumatic brain injury (TBI) or concussion. Headache is the most common manifestation, followed by insomnia, memory deficits, irritability, and dizziness. After acute trauma assessment and determination that the concussive injury is the sole issue, immediate management of these symptoms (eg, in the emergency department, military theater, or playing field) entails:

   • A comprehensive explanation to the patient/family of the nature of the TBI

   • A thorough explanation of the current symptoms (ie, how they are related to the concussion) and their management

   • A discussion of potential additional symptoms over the next 2 weeks

- A clear emphasis on the high likelihood of rapid symptom resolution and a return to fully normal functioning in the first 1 to 3 months

2. In 15%–30% of individuals who sustain a concussion (individuals with polytrauma tend to range on the high end), some of these symptoms may persist for longer than 3 months, a condition known as postconcussive syndrome (PCS). The array of difficulties seen with PCS may be physical (eg, headache, dizziness), cognitive (eg, difficulty concentrating, forgetfulness), emotional/behavioral (eg, irritability, poor frustration tolerance), and/or constitutional (eg, insomnia). Secondary symptoms can include light (photophobia) or sound (hyperaccussis) sensitivity, a depressed mood, and fatigue. No specific acute injury marker (ie, biomarker, imaging finding, initial symptom complex) has been consistently demonstrated to predict for a propensity to develop PCS; however, individuals with polytrauma (ie, TBI plus a significant secondary injury or medical disorder related to the initial trauma) are more likely to develop it. While individuals with PCS are still more likely to have progressive resolution of symptoms with a return to baseline (or near baseline) symptomatically, functionally, and by all testing at 1 year postinjury, these individuals should be managed with an interdisciplinary team approach. An interdisciplinary team of experienced professionals, with specific knowledge, training, and experience with individuals with PCS, should evaluate and manage all aspects of the individual's needs in collaboration with his/her primary care clinician.

3. There is no specific treatment for PCS itself, since it does not have an single underlying cause (ie, location in the brain or etiology of injury to brain); however, symptoms

can be treated. Extensive education is needed to explain the layers of issues often present, to dispel misinformation often given, and to assist the patient (and family) to begin the prolonged recovery process. Specific symptom management is identical to the care for these symptoms in the non-PCS population, including medications for headache or insomnia, structured therapy to decrease pain and enhance flexibility, a return to exercise, behavioral therapy, and work/school. While a return to baseline by 1 year postinjury is seen in 95% of civilians and more than 85% of service members, even in those individuals whose symptoms and the diagnoses of PCS may not disappear, a return to a productive and meaningful life is likely with deliberate and consistent care and full engagement of the individual in self-care and wellness.

Postconcussive Syndrome

Assessment

An interdisciplinary team of experienced professionals, with specific knowledge, training, and experience with individuals with PCS should evaluate and manage all aspects of the individual's needs in collaboration with their primary care clinician.

Physical, cognitive, and behavioral symptoms commonly occur acutely after mild TBI or concussion.

After acute trauma assessment and determination that the concussive injury is the sole issue, immediate management of these symptoms (eg, in the emergency department, military theater, or playing field) entails a thorough explanation to the patient/family about the nature and management of TBI, as well as potential additional symptoms over the next 2 weeks, and the likelihood of symptom resolution in 1–3 months.

Precautions

15%–30% of individuals who sustain a concussion will have symptoms that persist for longer than 3 months, or postconcussive syndrome (PCS).

Management

There is no specific treatment for PCS itself, since it does not have a single underlying lesion (ie, location in the brain or etiology of injury to brain) except avoiding overstimulation.

Extensive education is needed to explain the layers of issues often present, to dispel misinformation often given, and to assist the patient (and family) to begin the prolonged recovery process.

Specific symptom management is identical to the care for these symptoms in the non-PCS population, including medications for headache or insomnia, structured therapy to decrease pain and enhance flexibility, a return to exercise, behavioral therapy, and work/school.

Postdeployment

Syndrome in

Combat-Related TBI

1. Ninety percent of individuals with mild traumatic brain injury (TBI) from combat-related polytrauma have one or more significant concomitant disorders (most commonly chronic musculoskeletal pain, posttraumatic stress disorder [PTSD], depression and substance abuse) that increase the persistence of postconcussive syndrome (PCS), delay functional recovery and return to work, and may be associated with long-term disability and even cognitive decline (eg, chronic traumatic encephalopathy). This condition is known as postdeployment syndrome (PDS). Individuals with PDS are more likely to have had multiple combat tours with multiple concussive events, have had a delay in initial diagnosis

with associated delay in care and management, and usually receive considerable ongoing medical and psychological care.

2. As with traditional civilian PCS, the array of difficulties seen with PDS may be physical (eg, headache, dizziness), cognitive (eg, difficulty concentrating), emotional/behavioral (eg, irritability), and/or constitutional (eg, insomnia). Additionally, significant ongoing psychological distress, including suicidality, is not uncommon in this population. PDS is frequently mis- or underdiagnosed, with patients being seen by a series of different specialists (often without coordinated care) and receiving an array of diagnoses and treatments. As with concussion itself (as well as chronic pain, PTSD, depression, substance abuse, and many conditions seen in health care), there is no single biomarker (eg, blood or urine test), imaging study, or paper and pencil (neuropsychological) test for PDS. An interdisciplinary team of experienced professionals, ideally with specific knowledge, training, and experience with military and veteran populations, should assess and manage all aspects of the individual's needs in collaboration with his/her primary care clinician.

3. There is no specific treatment for PDS itself, since it does not have a single underlying cause; however, symptoms can be treated. Extensive education is needed to explain the layers of issues often present, to dispel misinformation often given, and to assist the patient (and family) to begin the prolonged recovery process. Specific symptom management is identical to the care for these symptoms in the non-PDS population, including medications for headache or insomnia, structured therapy to decrease pain and enhance flexibility, a return

to exercise, behavioral therapy, and work/school. While all symptoms and diagnoses of PDS may not disappear, a return to a productive and meaningful life is likely with deliberate and consistent care and full engagement of individuals in their wellness.

Postdeployment Syndrome

Assessment

An interdisciplinary team of experienced health professionals, with specific knowledge, training, and experience with individuals with PDS, should evaluate and manage all aspects of the individual's needs in collaboration with primary care clinicians.

Precautions

Ninety percent of individuals with mild TBI from combat-related polytrauma have one or more significant concomitant disorders that increase the persistence of postconcussive syndrome, delay functional recovery and return to work and may be associated with long-term disability and even cognitive decline.

Management

There is no specific treatment for PDS itself, since it does not have a single underlying cause; however, symptoms can be treated.

Extensive education is needed to explain the layers of issues often present, to dispel misinformation often given, and to assist the patient (and family) to begin the prolonged recovery process.

Specific symptom management is identical to the care for these symptoms in the non-PDS population, including medications for headache or insomnia, structured therapy to decrease pain and enhance flexibility, and a return to exercise, behavioral therapy, and work/school.

While all symptoms of PDS may not disappear, a return to a productive and meaningful life is likely with deliberate and consistent care and full engagement of individuals in their wellness.

Headaches

1. Headaches of some type are reported by 75% and incapacitates 10% of all Americans annually. Headaches are the most common symptom reported by individuals after polytrauma, and when a mild traumatic brain injury (TBI) has been experienced, more than 90% report difficulty with headaches. Importantly, headaches can also be associated with depression, posttraumatic stress disorder (PTSD), insomnia, anxiety disorder, and many other systemic physical and psychological disorders. A headache that begins within 2 weeks of a concussion is considered to be related to the injury and is labeled a posttraumatic headache (PTHA). If a PTHA continues for more than 8 weeks it is considered a chronic PTHA, which occurs in nearly 50% of combat injured individuals with polytrauma.

2. The majority of headaches after polytrauma will lessen in intensity and frequency after a few weeks and can be simply managed. In addition to standard dose over-the-counter headache medications (eg, acetaminophen), attention to the following will enhance recovery: normalizing sleep patterns,

maintaining a simple and balanced diet (eg, chocolate may worsen headaches, excessive caffeine use or caffeine withdrawal may worsen headaches), performing several times daily stress relaxation exercises, performing several times daily shoulder and neck stretching, performing daily aerobic and movement exercise, and returning to purposeful activity (eg, hobby, work, volunteering). Headaches that are recalcitrant to these approaches will benefit by further categorization and focused treatments.

3. Tension headaches are the most common nontraumatic headaches and may be seen in 25% of polytrauma patients with headaches. They are usually bilateral head pain, nonthrobbing in nature, mild to moderate and steady in intensity, and not worsened by physical activity. While these headaches usually respond to the basic interventions, if recalcitrant, clinicians may consider tricyclic antidepressants (TCAs; eg, nortriptyline) as a second-line medication. Selective serotoninergic-norepinephrine reuptake inhibitors (SNRIs) and anticonvulsants (eg, topiramate, gabapentin) may also be considered.

4. Migraine headaches are common (10% of all Americans annually) in individuals without trauma exposure, but more common (25% of polytrauma patients) after concussion, where they are referred to as posttraumatic migraines. Migraine headaches usually begin gradually in the daytime with a mild, dull, deep, steady pain across the entire head or in a specific area (usually the front of the head or eyes) and evolve to an increasing amount of severe, throbbing pain. Some migraines are preceded by a strange sensation (aura), usually visual (flash of light/scotoma, light sensitivity/photophobia). Migraines can be brought on by medications (risperidol, nitroglycerin) and menstruation. Anticonvulsants and beta-blockers may prevent migraine headaches and can be considered in patients with frequent recurrences. Botulinum injections into the muscles around the neck and skull may also be used to temporarily weaken these muscles (for 2–6 months) and prevent recurrence. Triptan and ergotamine medications are used to abort an impending migraine headaches.

5. Cervicogenic headaches are the most common headache seen after polytrauma with concussion and are also associated with whiplash injuries of the head and neck seen in both combat and civilian trauma. While elements of both tension and migraine headaches may be seen in these patients, cervicogenic headache should be the diagnosis when there are specific soft tissue areas (muscle, tendon) that initiate or worsen the pain when pressed or stretched. Headaches are associated with prolonged postures or certain neck movements. Pain radiates upward from the neck to the head and specific regions of the skull. Muscles are either tender or can generate the headache when compressed. Cluster headaches will respond well with the basic headache approach outlined above, oftentimes accompanied by scheduled dosing of nonsteroidal anti-inflammatories (NSAIDs) for 2 to 4 weeks. Botulinum toxin may be considered for persistent headaches.

6. Other causes of PTHA are rare, but include cluster headaches (autonomic symptoms associated with severe eye pain), neuropathic headaches (extreme sensitivity or allodynia of the face), chronic daily headaches (nonspecific head pain 15 days per month for 3 months), primary exertional headaches (throbbing bilateral head pain that occurs during or immediately after exercise), and cerebral spinal fluid (CSF)-related headaches (intense headaches that are relieved by lying flat and are associated with skull fracture or other causes of CSF leak).

Headaches

Assessment

A headache that begins within 2 weeks of a head trauma is considered to be related to the injury and is labeled a posttraumatic headache (PTHA).

A PTHA that continues for more than 8 weeks is considered a chronic PTHA.

Precautions

Headaches of some type are reported by 75% of the uninjured population, 90% of individuals with mTBI, and incapacitates 10% of all Americans annually.

Management

The majority of headaches after polytrauma will lessen in intensity and frequency after a few weeks and can be simply managed.

In addition to standard dose over-the-counter medications, attention to the following will enhance recovery:

- Normalizing sleep patterns
- Maintaining a simple and balanced diet
- Performing several times daily stress relaxation exercises
- Performing several times daily shoulder and neck stretching
- Performing daily aerobic and movement exercise
- Returning to purposeful activity

Headaches that are recalcitrant to these approaches will benefit by further categorization and focused treatments.

- Tension—consider nortriptyline
- Migraine—consider anticonvulsants or beta-blockers
- Cervicogenic—consider stretching program

Insomnia

1. Sleep disturbances, either too little (insomnia) or too much (hypersomnia), are a common complaint with a whole range of physical (eg, acute or chronic pain, obesity, brain injury) and psychological (eg, posttraumatic stress disorder [PTSD], depression) disorders and may also been seen in otherwise healthy individuals. Servicemembers who have been deployed into a military theater frequently experience insomnia for as long as 3 months after they return to their homes due to the trauma and stresses of war. Individuals who have suffered polytrauma experience insomnia (and less commonly hypersomnia) frequently, especially if they have sustained a brain injury.

2. Irregular, insufficient (<7 hours/night) or otherwise inadequately restful sleep alone can cause a range of difficulties, including headache, bodily pain, dizziness, mood disturbances (irritability, mood swings, sadness, euphoria, anxiety), inattention, poor concentration, and memory loss. Restorative sleep includes a series of alternating phases (usually 5 or more) of the relaxed nonrapid eye movement

(non-REM) phase, usually 75% of all sleep, and the active REM phase. A focused program of sleep hygiene with improved rest can markedly improve many symptoms that commonly accompany polytrauma. Elements of good sleep hygiene that can help restore restful sleep (ie, alternating REM and non-REM phases) include:

- Treating any medical conditions (eg, sleep apnea)
- Performing at least 45 minutes of conditional exercise or activity daily (at least 2 hours before sleeping)
- Not eating at least 2 hours before sleeping
- Using the bathroom 30 minutes or less before sleeping
- Avoiding any stimulants (caffeine, energy drinks, tobacco) at least 4 hours before sleeping
- Spending the final 30 minutes before sleeping in a low stimuli (light, noise), relaxed (soothing music/sounds, meditating, deep breathing) environment
- Avoiding daytime naps and sedating medications/alcohol
- Establishing a regular sleep and wake schedule

3. Sleep apnea is a sleep disorder characterized by abnormal pauses (apnea) in breathing or instances of abnormally low breathing (hypopnea), during sleep. Each pause in breathing can last from at least 10 seconds to minutes, and may occur 5 to 30 times or more an hour. These difficulties may be due to central (brain) causes, obstructive (mouth and upper airway) causes, or a combination of both. Purely central causes are extremely rare and the very common obstructive causes are frequently associated with snoring. While most individuals are not aware they are having these episodes, they may be witnessed by their sleeping partner, or the individual may complain of fatigue, poor attention, and slowed reaction time. Treatment entails avoiding sedating medications and alcohol (these may overly relax the oral/

pharyngeal muscles), weight loss (improving the oral/ pharyngeal spaces), and side sleeping. Oral appliances (nighttime mouth/jaw braces) to open the airway may have some effect. Continuous positive airway pressure (CPAP) delivered via a face mask is used to splint open the airway via pressurized air. In recalcitrant sleep apnea surgical interventions have been utilized.

4. For patients who cannot be managed with a comprehensive program of sleep hygiene (and do not have sleep apnea), medications are often helpful for short-term correction insomnia. The most appropriate medications are nonaddictive, have rapid onset of action, and no other systemic effects. The three most commonly used medications for simple insomnia are trazadone (50–200 mg 30 minutes before sleep), zolpidem (5–10 mg 30 minutes before sleep), and eszopiclone (2–3 mg 30 minutes before sleep). For individuals with polytrauma who have insomnia and nightmares, prazosin (usually given in the morning and at night, in doses as high as 40 mg daily), and risperidol (1–2 mg at night) have been recommended. Importantly, over-the-counter (OTC) medications and herbals should be used with extreme caution and monitoring as their efficacy has not been proven and their specific ingredients are not always clearly indicated. Long-term use (>3 months) of any medications and the use of addictive (eg, benzodiazepines) medications are not recommended.

Insomnia

Assessment

Irregular, insufficient, or otherwise inadequately restful sleep alone can cause a range of difficulties, including headache, bodily pain, dizziness, mood disturbances (irritability, mood swings, sadness, euphoria, anxiety), inattention, poor concentration, and memory loss.

Restorative sleep includes a series of alternating phases (usually 5 or more) of the relaxed nonrapid eye movement (non-REM) phase, usually 75% of all sleep, and the active REM phase.

Precautions

Over-the-counter medications and herbals should be used with extreme caution and monitoring as their efficacy has not been proven and their specific ingredients are not always clearly indicated.

Long-term use (>3 months) of any medications and the use of addictive medications is not recommended.

Management

A focused program of sleep hygiene with improved rest can markedly improve many symptoms that commonly accompany polytrauma.

Three most commonly used medications for simple insomnia are trazadone (50–200 mg 30 minutes before sleep), zolpidem (5–10 mg 30 minutes before sleep), and eszopiclone (2–3 mg 30 minutes before sleep).

For individuals with polytrauma who have insomnia and nightmares, prazosin (usually given in the morning and at night, in doses as high as 40 mg daily) and risperidol (1–2 mg at night) are used.

Penetrating Brain Injuries

1. While the vast majority (>80%) of brain injuries associated with either civilian or combat polytrauma injury are mild in severity (alteration or loss of consciousness for <30 minutes and typically normal head computed tomography [CT] scan), injuries of greater severity do occur. Most of these injuries are of moderate severity (alteration or loss of consciousness for up to 24 hours, abnormal CT scan of the head) and a very small percentage is labeled as severe (loss of consciousness for more than 24 hours). A very small portion of these severe injuries are categorized as "open" or "penetrating," and tend to be the most severe and significant of all injuries.

2. A penetrating head injury, or open head (brain) injury, is a brain injury in which the dura mater (the outer layer of the meninges or covering of the brain) is breached. Penetrating

injury can be caused by high-velocity projectiles (eg, bullets, fragments from explosives), objects of lower velocity (eg, knives), or bone fragments from a skull fracture that are driven into the brain. Head injuries caused by penetrating trauma are serious medical emergencies and may cause permanent disability or death due to the initial trauma or the secondary medical conditions that may develop.

3. The highest-velocity injuries tend to have the worst associated damage with associated high rates of chronic disability or death. Injuries that cross the midline, involve the brainstem, or perforate the skull in two places (ie, have an exit wound) have the worst prognosis. While many components of penetrating injury are similar to the devastation caused by severe closed head injury, there are additional immediate, acute, and chronic effects. The immediate effects of penetrating injuries involve direct brain trauma, bleeding with local injury, and elevated risk of vasospasm (with associated ischemia), and acute brain swelling. Acute effects of penetrating injury include a marked elevated risk for infection, cerebral spinal fluid (CSF) leakage and obstructive hydrocephalus (related to edema, blood products in the subarachnoid space, and foreign bodies/bone in the CSF circulation). The major chronic effect of penetrating head injury is an elevated risk for posttraumatic epilepsy (recurrent seizures).

4. Treatment for individuals with open or penetrating brain injury, after establishing cardiovascular and pulmonary stability, entails acute debridement of damaged brain tissue, removal of skull/missile fragments, and evacuation of blood. Close surveillance for

the common effects of the injury are combined with traditional medical and rehabilitation efforts. Often skull closure must be accomplished with a delayed (ie, 6+ weeks) cranioplasty, if a skull defect is caused by the injury or warranted (ie, craniectomy) by the injury management.

Disorders of

Consciousness

1. Disorders of consciousness (DOC) result from medical conditions that inhibit self-awareness and purposeful activity. DOC include minimally conscious state (MCS), vegetative state (VS), and persistent vegetative state (PVS). Conditions in which individuals have awareness but poor ability to interact with the environment or make their intent known, such as locked-in syndrome and akinetic mutism, are not true DOC but are often mistaken for it. While other conditions may cause a moderate deterioration (eg, dementia and delirium) or transient interruption (eg, grand mal and petit mal seizures) of consciousness, they are not included in this category.

2. Individuals who sustain polytrauma with severe traumatic brain injury (TBI) are often initially in a comatose or VS (no awareness of their environment and unable to follow commands). More than 90% of individuals who

are initially in coma will rapidly or gradually improve in the first 4 weeks after injury and begin to meaningfully interact with the environment. Those patients who improve but do so slowly are labeled as being in MCS, with intermittent periods of awareness and wakefulness and a display of some meaningful behavior. If patients remain in a VS, they are classified as in a PVS. In PVS, the patient has sleep-wake cycles, but lacks awareness and only displays reflexive and nonpurposeful behavior. It is a diagnosis of some uncertainty in that it deals with a syndrome. This diagnosis is classified as a permanent vegetative state after 1 year of being in a VS.

3. While an adequately functioning cerebral cortex (particularly the frontal lobes) is needed to effectively sense and interact with the environment, the brainstem reticular activating system (RAS) is needed to maintain consciousness. Made up of a system of acetylcholine-producing neurons, the ascending track, or ascending reticular activating system (ARAS), works to arouse and wake up the brain from the reticular function, through the thalamus, and then finally to the cerebral cortex. A failure in ARAS functioning may then lead to a coma. It is therefore necessary to investigate the integrity of the bilateral cerebral cortices, as well as that of the RAS in a comatose patient.

4. While a number of medications to provide activation may be considered, there is little evidence that they have any effect. These medications include certain antidepressants, amantadine, bromocriptine, and methylphenidate. Until these patients "awaken" from their PVS to a level of MCS, there's little support for any of these agents.

5. In addition to optimizing care (eg, monitoring for hydrocephalus, seizures, infection, hypoxia, metabolic,

and endocrinologic abnormalities) to allow for natural recovery after injury, rehabilitative interventions to facilitate improvement from a DOC include normalizing sleep-wake cycles through appropriate sleep hygiene, eliminating distracting background environment stimulation (eg, television, cluttered rooms, excess light), establishing a schedule with periods of focused and appropriate stimuli (eg, nondistracting environment, specific tasking, no sedating medications) alternating with controlled periods of rest, and eliminating medications that may be sedating or confusing. Superior nursing care is critical to the short- and long-term recovery from a DOC. While specialized rehabilitation therapists should be involved in the initial assessment, establishment of individualized stimulation programs (eg, periodic sitting or standing, tactile stimulation, teaching family to provide repeated vocal stimulation), and periodic reevaluation, the 24 hour/day physical and psychological care of these individuals provided by nursing (and families) is the key element in a positive recovery. Initial research in the polytrauma populations has suggested a more than 60% chance of awakening from PVS, so meticulous and consistent nursing care is crucial in allowing for the eventual rehabilitation of patients who emerge from a DOC.

Disorders of Consciousness

Assessment

Comatose or vegetative state (VS): no awareness of environment and unable to follow commands.

Minimal conscious state (MCS): intermittent periods of awareness and wakefulness and a display of some meaningful behavior.

Persistent vegetative state (PVS): has sleep-wake cycles, but lack of awareness and only displays reflexive and nonpurposeful behavior.

Permanent vegetative state indicates ≥1 year of coma.

↓

Precautions

More than 90% of individuals who are initially in coma will rapidly or gradually improve in the first 4 weeks after injury and begin to meaningfully interact with the environment.

↓

Management

There is little evidence that medications have any impact until patients have "awakened" to a level of MCS.

Optimizing care (eg, monitoring for hydrocephalus, seizures, infection, hypoxia, metabolic, and endocrinologic abnormalities) to allow for natural recovery is the main intervention.

Rehabilitative interventions to facilitate improvement from disorders of consciousness (DOC) include normalizing sleep-wake cycles through appropriate sleep hygiene, eliminating distracting background environment stimulation, establishing a schedule with periods of focused and appropriate stimuli alternating with controlled periods of rest, and eliminating medications that may be sedating or confusing.

Superior nursing care is critical to the short- and long-term recovery from a DOC.

Posttraumatic Seizures

1. Posttraumatic seizures (PTS) are transient symptoms of abnormal excessive or synchronous neuronal activity in the brain that may manifest as a wild thrashing movement (tonic-clonic seizure) or as mild as a brief loss of awareness (absence seizure), and are the result of acute or chronic damage to the brain from traumatic brain injury (TBI). PTS may be labeled as "immediate" (in the first 24 hours of injury), "acute" (from 24 hours to 7 days postinjury), or "late" (more than 1 week postinjury). A person with posttraumatic epilepsy (PTE) suffers repeated late PTS. PTE is estimated to constitute 5% of all cases of epilepsy and over 20% of cases of symptomatic epilepsy.

2. Immediate PTS are usually the result of acute alterations in the physiology of the brain and stress on the brain cells caused by hypoxia, metabolic abnormalities (usually low sodium), irritation from blood, medication effect, drug or alcohol withdrawal, or increased intracranial pressure. Once these irritants are removed or have resolved, there is no further risk for seizure and no long-term

elevated risk. This is probably also true for early PTS, although a clear causal factor should be identified before this is assumed. Extensive research strongly supports the usage of therapeutic dosing of anticonvulsant medications (either phenytoin or carbamazepine) for the first week postinjury (but not longer). On the other hand, late PTS is more likely related to a focal area of brain injury that is producing the neuronal discharge, which may recover or may persist. Individuals who develop late PTS should be treated with therapeutic anticonvulsants for at least 12 months to attempt to "quiet" this injured brain region and reduce the risk of PTE. While there may be other factors that increase the likelihood of developing PTE (eg, penetrating brain injury, age older than 60, hydrocephalus), there has been no research to support the efficacy of ongoing use of anticonvulsants in these patients. Similarly, there is no value in using electroencephalography (EEG) or neuroimaging to track or categorize patients for PTE risk.

3. Individuals who sustain polytrauma with mild TBI have demonstrated a higher incidence of "nonepileptic seizures." Nonepileptic seizures are paroxysmal events that mimic a seizure but do not involve abnormal, rhythmic discharges of cortical neurons. They are caused by either physiological (eg, low blood sugar, migraine, hypoxia) or psychological (eg, stress, anxiety) conditions. While physiologic causes should be thoroughly evaluated, the most common cause in individuals with polytrauma has been linked with secondary psychological conditions. Treatment should focus on education, counseling, cognitive behavioral therapy, sleep hygiene, and a focus on return to productive activity.

4. In addition to appropriate medications and management by neurology specialty, individuals with PTE should be extensively counseled on prohibited activities (if their epilepsy is not controlled), such as driving, use of heavy machinery, being on ladders, bathing, and swimming, and on the importance of having a "buddy" for these activities if they have had good control but have had a seizure in the past 5 years. In the United States, most states require at least 6 months of seizure-free activity before the legal return to driving. If cognitive or motoric deficits persist after PTS or as a result of medications to control the seizures, then a formal driving test or driver's rehabilitation is recommended.

Posttraumatic Seizures

Assessment

Posttraumatic seizures (PTS) may be labeled:

- Immediate—in the first 24 hours of injury
- Acute—from 24 hours to 7 days postinjury
- Late—more than 1 week postinjury

Precautions

There is not sufficient evidence to support the clinical usage of EEG or neuroimaging to track or categorize patients for PTE risk.

Individuals who sustain polytrauma with mild TBI have demonstrated a higher incidence of "nonepileptic seizures."

Management

The first line management of persistent PTS (or epilepsy) is appropriate medications and management by a neurology specialist.

Research supports the usage of therapeutic dosing of anticonvulsant medications (either phenytoin or carbamazepine) for the first week postinjury to prevent the occurrence of late PTS.

Individuals with PTE should be extensively counseled on prohibited activities (if their epilepsy is not controlled), such as driving, use of heavy machinery, being on ladders, bathing, and swimming, and on the importance of having a "buddy" for these activities if they have had good control but have had a seizure in the past 5 years.

In the United States, most states require at least 6 months of seizure-free activity before the legal return to driving.

Craniotomy/

Craniectomy/

Cranioplasty

1. A craniotomy is surgical hole made in the skull and dura to evacuate blood (eg, subdural hematoma) or cerebral spinal fluid (eg, with increased intracranial pressure), or to allow access to monitor the brain (eg, pressure, fluid chemistry) or perform a procedure (eg, brain biopsy, deep brain stimulation). While it increases the risk for intracranial infection and late posttraumatic seizures (a week of anticonvulsant prophylaxis is recommended), there are otherwise few long-term sequelae and no specific precautions required afterward.

2. A craniectomy is the surgical removal of a section of the skull. Related to polytrauma injury, this is typically done following severe traumatic brain injury (TBI) to evacuate

significant amounts of blood, to debride brain tissue (usually following penetrating head injury), and/or to rapidly alleviate elevated intracranial pressure. Owing to the propensity for postcraniectomy intracranial swelling or, with many penetrating injuries, to there being insufficient skull bone to adequately close the skull deficit, the craniectomy deficit is typically left open (with closure of the dura). Viable skull that is removed is either frozen or placed in the patient's abdominal cavity (where it survives well) after being sterilized. While this results in a significant cosmetic deficit and may result in an increase in localized headache (particularly with rapid head movements) for 2 to 4 weeks, temporary cranial defects are well tolerated by patients and do not delay rehabilitation efforts. All patients with craniectomy deficits must wear a protective helmet (eg, hockey or bicycle-type helmet) when out of bed.

3. Cranioplasty is the surgical repair of a skull deficit or deformity, and in polytrauma patients with skull deficit after TBI this is typically performed 6 to 12 months after the initial injury. Given the higher incidence of intracranial infection in individuals with polytrauma (due to the higher incidence of open head injury, foreign bodies, and contaminated wounds on the battlefield), cranioplasties are performed significantly later compared with civilian injury. Individuals who do not have adequate skull tissue frozen/stored to fill the defect use custom-molded skull prostheses. Typically the surgical closure with cranioplasty is sufficient to allow for removal of the protective helmet immediately postoperatively.

Hydrocephalus

1. Hydrocephalus entails an abnormal accumulation of cerebrospinal fluid (CSF) in the ventricles, or cavities, of the brain that is common with severe traumatic brain injury (TBI) after polytrauma. The clinical presentation of hydrocephalus varies based on how long it has been present. Acute dilatation of the ventricular system is more likely to manifest with the nonspecific signs and symptoms (somnolence, headache, vomiting, seizures, papilledema) of increased intracranial pressure. Acute elevated intracranial pressure may result in uncal and/or cerebellar tonsil herniation, with resulting life-threatening brainstem compression. By contrast chronic dilatation may have a more insidious onset with a classic triad of symptoms of gait instability, urinary incontinence, and dementia.

2. Hydrocephalus can be caused by impaired CSF flow, reabsorption, or excessive CSF production. The most common cause of hydrocephalus with polytrauma is CSF flow obstruction, hindering the free passage of CSF through the ventricular system and subarachnoid space

(eg, obstruction of the interventricular foramina—foramina of Monro secondary to hemorrhages or infection). Based on its underlying mechanisms, hydrocephalus can be classified into communicating and noncommunicating (obstructive).

3. Communicating hydrocephalus, also known as non-obstructive hydrocephalus, is caused by impaired CSF resorption in the absence of any CSF flow obstruction between the ventricles and subarachnoid space. This may be due to functional impairment, caused by subarachnoid hemorrhage, or infectious/inflammatory debris, of the arachnoidal granulations, which are located along the superior sagittal sinus and is the site of CSF resorption back into the venous system. Noncommunicating hydrocephalus, or obstructive hydrocephalus, is caused by a CSF flow obstruction, ultimately preventing CSF from flowing into the subarachnoid space either due to external compression (eg, generalized brain edema) or intraventricular mass lesions (eg, blood, bone fragment, foreign body).

4. Normal pressure hydrocephalus (NPH) is a particular form of communicating hydrocephalus, characterized by enlarged cerebral ventricles, with only intermittently elevated CSF pressure. The diagnosis of NPH can be established only with the help of continuous intraventricular pressure recordings (over 24 hours or even longer), since more often than not instant measurements yield normal pressure values. Dynamic compliance studies may be also helpful. Altered compliance (elasticity) of the ventricular walls, as well as increased viscosity of the CSF, may play a role in the pathogenesis of NPH.

5. Hydrocephalus ex vacuo also refers to an enlargement of cerebral ventricles and subarachnoid spaces, and is usually due to brain atrophy from aging or dementia or post-TBI. As opposed to hydrocephalus, this is a compensatory enlargement of the CSF spaces in response to brain parenchyma loss—it is not the result of increased CSF pressure.

Hydrocephalus

Assessment

Acute hydrocephalus can be detected by individual or serial CT scans of the brain.

Chronic hydrocephalus requires continuous intraventricular pressure recordings (over 24 hours or even longer), since instant, individual measurements often yield normal pressure values. Dynamic compliance studies may be also helpful.

Precautions

Acute hydrocephalus presents with the nonspecific signs and symptoms (somnolence, headache, vomiting, seizures, papilledema) of increased intracranial pressure (IICP).

Chronic hydrocephalus has an insidious onset with a classic triad of symptoms of gait instability, urinary incontinence, and dementia.

Management

Persistent (acute or chronic) hydrocephalus must be treated with CSF drainage to relieve the pressure.

Implanted CSF shunts need to be calibrated to the CSF imbalance and often must be adjusted (downward) as the patient improves from injury.

Neuroendocrinologic Abnormalities

1. Neuroendocrine dysfunction following polytrauma has been well-defined for individuals with severe traumatic brain injury (TBI), particularly those who have a significant duration with a disorder of consciousness (coma), but has also been well described for those with mild TBI/concussion. TBIs that result in either direct (bleeding, penetrating trauma) or indirect (pressure) injury to the deeper, subcortical structures of the brain may cause temporary or chronic dysfunction of the hypothalamic–pituitary–adrenal (HPA) axis, which regulates neuroendocrine functioning. In all individuals with severe TBI and in those with persistent symptoms after less severe injury (eg, postdeployment syndrome, postconcussive syndrome), an evaluation of neuroendocrine functioning is recommended.

2. The HPA axis, also known as the limbic-HPA axis and the HPA-gonadotropic axis, is a complex set of

direct influences and feedback interactions among the hypothalamus, the pituitary gland, and the adrenal glands. The interactions among these organs constitute the HPA axis, a major part of the neuroendocrine system that controls reactions to stress and regulates many body processes, including digestion, the immune system, mood and emotions, sexuality, and energy storage and expenditure. Anatomical connections among brain areas such as the amygdala, hippocampus, and hypothalamus facilitate activation of the HPA axis. Sensory information arriving at the lateral aspect of the amygdala is processed and conveyed to the central nucleus, which projects to several parts of the brain involved in responses to fear, including posttraumatic stress disorder (PTSD). At the hypothalamus, fear-signaling impulses activate both the sympathetic nervous system and the modulating systems of the HPA axis.

3. The hypothalamus is located below the thalamus, just above the brainstem, and is made up of a number of nuclei that control endocrinologic functions of the body linked with neurologic function. Adjacent to the pituitary, it is an endocrine gland that sits in a small, bony cavity at the base of the brain (the sella tursica) and whose secretions control the other endocrine glands and influence growth, metabolism, and maturation. The adenohypophysis is the anterior lobe of the pituitary gland, producing and secreting several peptide hormones that regulate many physiological processes including stress, growth, and reproduction, including the functioning of the thyroid gland. The neurohypophysis is the posterior lobe of the pituitary gland, responsible for the release of oxytocin and antidiuretic hormone (ADH), also called vasopressin. The hypothalamus controls the regulation of

cortisol-releasing hormone (CRH) influenced by stress, physical activity, illness, blood levels of cortisol, and the sleep/wake cycle (circadian rhythm). The HPA axis controls development, reproduction, and aging in animals. The hypothalamus produces gonadotropin-releasing hormone (GnRH). The anterior portion of the pituitary gland produces luteinizing hormone (LH) and follicle-stimulating hormone (FSH), and the gonads produce estrogen and testosterone.

4. Individuals who have had mild TBI with polytrauma and who have also had significant other physical (eg, pain, fracture, soft tissue injury) or psychological (eg, PTSD, generalized anxiety disorder) stressors may develop abnormalities of their neuroendocrine functioning/HPA axis due to these excessive or persisting stresses. For example, the HPA axis will increase production of cortisol as part of the alarm reactions, facilitating an adaptive phase of a general adaptation syndrome in which alarm reactions including the immune response are suppressed, allowing the body to attempt countermeasures. This will facilitate the release of glucocorticoids to help modulate these stress reactions, but when these stresses persist or are perceived to be persisting, glucocorticoid excess can be damaging. Atrophy of the hippocampus in humans and animals exposed to severe stress is believed to be caused by prolonged exposure to high concentrations of glucocorticoids. These deficiencies of the hippocampus may result in a reduction in both day-to-day memory and the memory resources available to help a body formulate appropriate reactions to current or future stresses.

5. Evaluation of the HPA axis can be challenging due to its diverse functioning and the manifold factors that

can influence it. These factors can include the duration of hospitalization, nutritional status, medications, medical status (eg, presence of infections), activity level, secondary medical conditions, psychological status, and others. Screening of all individuals with severe initial injury should be considered when they are transitioned from acute medical care (usually 2–6 weeks postinjury) and should include testing for thyroid function, growth hormone, serum/urine cortisol, serum/urine sodium, and sex hormones (testosterone, estrogen). Individuals with persistent symptoms after polytrauma/concussion that are not responding to symptom-based care should be tested at 3 months. Collaboration with an experienced endocrinologist is encouraged prior to hormonal supplementation due to the challenges with interpreting "abnormal" tests and the numerous hormonal interactions.

Neuroendocrinologic Abnormalities

Assessment

Neuroendocrine screening of all individuals with severe initial TBI should be considered when they are transitioned from acute medical care (usually 2–6 weeks postinjury) and should include testing for thyroid function, growth hormone, serum/urine cortisol, serum/urine sodium, and sex hormones (testosterone, estrogen).

Individuals with persistent symptoms after polytrauma/concussion who are not responding to symptom-based care should be tested at 3 months.

Precautions

Individuals who have had mild TBI with polytrauma and who have also had significant other physical or psychological stressors may develop abnormalities of their neuroendocrine functioning/hypothalamic–pituitary–adrenal (HPA) axis due to these excessive or persisting stresses.

Management

Collaboration with an experienced endocrinologist is encouraged prior to hormonal supplementation due to the challenges with interpreting "abnormal" tests and the numerous hormonal interactions.

Geriatric and Aging Issues

1. While the vast majority of injuries in polytrauma occur in the young to middle-aged populations, it is important to be aware of unique issues related to injury in the older population, and to also understand the effect of aging in patients who sustained polytrauma. In civilian brain injury, older adults are the second most commonly affected population, so an understanding of these issues will be relevant to this cohort as well.

2. Polytrauma injuries that occur to older adults are more often fatal and will usually result in a greater degree of functional impairment than younger adults, owing to the greater prevalence of secondary medical and disabling conditions and the resulting decrease in physiologic and functional reserve. Older adults are more likely to require longer acute and rehabilitation care to address the greater severity of injury/disability and the slower

recovery seen. Additionally, older adults are more likely to require long-term care (at home or in an institution) after or instead of inpatient rehabilitation care. Note, however, that research has demonstrated that a significant proportion of older adults can tolerate and participate in intensive rehabilitation programs and will make functional gains.

3. Special attention needs to be given to the care of older adults with polytrauma and traumatic brain injury (TBI) to optimize recovery and to be sensitive to their needs. This includes a greater awareness of and more in-depth knowledge and use of rehabilitation interventions to address:
   - Their underlying and acute comorbid conditions, which tend to be of greater number and complexity
   - The effects of polypharmacy and the impact of central-acting medications on brain functioning
   - The higher incidence of a decrease in the special senses (hearing, vision, taste, sensation) with needed accommodations
   - The mild to moderate decline in cognition, reaction time, balance and motor function
   - The decrease in exercise and activity tolerance
   - The social and cultural differences that likely exist between the patient and clinicians (eg, multigenerational issues)
   - The preinjury and altered postinjury family dynamics
   - The specifics of Medicare and Medicaid

4. While there is limited research clearly outlining the specifics of aging with polytrauma and TBI, many of the considerations for the acute management of older adults can be applied to individuals who sustained their injuries during middle age and are now facing challenges related to "normal" aging. For individuals who have

persistent functional deficits after TBI, independence is likely to become more challenging as the physiologic and functional reserve deficits that accompany aging occur. These individuals will benefit from periodic reevaluation and care by rehabilitation specialists, and their families will likely benefit from ongoing education, support and, if needed, respite. For individuals without significant functional deficits (eg, a history of concussion), it is unclear if there are specific rehabilitative interventions (eg, structured therapy, staged inpatient care) to enhance abilities, however it has been shown that encouraging healthy nutrition with weight management, avoiding tobacco usage, using alcohol in moderation, regular conditioning and functionally focused exercise (eg, walking), consistent primary medical care, engagement in cognitive stimulating activities (eg, work, volunteerism, hobbies) alternating with restorative rest, and maintaining rich social contacts (eg, family, friends, groups) will allow for optimal cognitive, behavioral, and physical functioning in elders. A focus on long-term prevention of repeat injury (eg, fall prevention) and other safety issues (eg, periodically monitoring driving abilities, assessing the ability to live alone) is also an important aspect of chronic management. There is limited evidence to suggest that single or multiple polytrauma injuries or concussion will ultimately result in degeneration of brain function (ie, dementia); however, if there is a subpopulation that is at higher risk for this, a focus on comprehensive health and wellness is likely the most appropriate approach to their long-term care as well.

Dementia and Brain Injury

1. There is limited but growing evidence to suggest that there may be a subpopulation of individuals with multiple concussions or more severe initial traumatic brain injury (TBI) who will ultimately develop degeneration of brain function (ie, dementia). The multiple factors that may contribute to brain degeneration over a long period of time (eg, genetics, cardiovascular disease, alcohol and substance use, tobacco usage, chronic psychological disorders, limited cognitive stimulation, physical inactivity, "normal" aging) and the overlap of the more common dementing and degenerative disorders (eg, Alzheimer's disease, Parkinson's disease) need to be carefully considered before any conclusions about the uniqueness of this condition may be made. However, many believe that there is a discrete disorder, labeled chronic traumatic encephalopathy (CTE), which is a progressive degenerative disease usually diagnosed postmortem in individuals with a history

of multiple concussions and other forms of head injury. While initially described more than 50 years ago in a small number of people and termed "dementia pugilistica," CTE has been most commonly found in professional athletes participating in American football, ice hockey, boxing, and other contact sports. It has also been found related to polytrauma with blast exposure and concussive injury. CTE manifests in brain tissue with the accumulation of tau protein ("tauopathy"). Individuals with CTE may show symptoms of dementia, such as memory loss, aggression, confusion, and depression, which may appear within months of the trauma or many decades later.

2. The primary pathological manifestations of CTE include a reduction in brain weight associated with atrophy of the frontal and temporal cortices and medial temporal lobe. The lateral ventricles and the third ventricle are often enlarged, with rare instances of dilation of the fourth ventricle. Other pathological manifestations of CTE include pallor of the substantia nigra and locus ceruleus, and atrophy of the olfactory bulbs, thalamus, mammillary bodies, brainstem, and cerebellum. As CTE progresses, there may be marked atrophy of the hippocampus, entorhinal cortex, and amygdala. On a microscopic scale the pathology includes neuronal loss, tau deposition, TAR DNA-binding protein 43 (TDP 43) beta-amyloid deposition, white matter changes, and other abnormalities. The tau deposition occurs as dense neurofibrillary tangles (NFT), neurites, and glial tangles, which are made up of astrocytes and other glial cells. Beta-amyloid deposition is an inconstant feature of CTE.

3. While the diagnosis of CTE is made postmortem, some common findings are medical histories with past traumatic

brain injuries and secondary symptoms that include disorientation, confusion, vertigo, headaches, poor judgment, overt dementia, slowed muscular movements, staggered gait, impeded speech, tremors, and deafness. Individuals suffering from CTE may also progress through three stages of the disease: (1) evidence of the neurologic and cognitive disturbances and psychotic symptoms, (2) exhibition of erratic behavior, memory loss, and the initial symptoms of Parkinson's disease, such as difficulty with balance and gait, and (3) frank dementia.

4. For individuals who have persistent physical and cognitive functional deficits after TBI, the development of degenerative processes is more likely. These individuals will benefit from periodic reevaluation and care by rehabilitation specialists, and their families will likely benefit from ongoing education, support, and, if needed, respite. For individuals without significant functional deficits (eg, a history of concussion) after injury, it is unclear if there are specific rehabilitative interventions (eg, structured therapy, staged inpatient care) to prevent CTE; however, in older adults in general it has been shown that encouraging healthy nutrition with weight management, avoiding tobacco usage, using alcohol in moderation, regular conditioning and functionally focused exercise (eg, walking), consistent primary medical care, engagement in cognitive stimulating activities (eg, work, volunteerism, hobbies) alternating with restorative rest, and maintaining rich social contacts (eg, family, friends, groups) will allow for optimal cognitive, behavioral, and physical functioning. A focus on long-term prevention of repeat injury (eg, fall prevention) and other safety issues (eg, periodically monitoring driving abilities, assessing

the ability to live alone) is also an important aspect of care. While at present, there is limited evidence to suggest that single or multiple polytrauma injuries or concussion will ultimately result in degeneration of brain function (ie, dementia), if there is a subpopulation that is at higher risk for this, a focus on their comprehensive health and wellness is likely the most appropriate approach to their long-term care as well.

Dementia and Brain Injury

Assessment

The diagnosis of chronic traumatic encephalopathy (CTE) is made postmortem, but common findings are medical histories with past traumatic brain injuries and secondary symptoms that include disorientation, confusion, vertigo, headaches, poor judgment, overt dementia, slowed muscular movements, staggered gait, impeded speech, tremors, and deafness.

The primary pathological manifestations of CTE include a reduction in brain weight, associated with atrophy of the frontal and temporal cortices and medial temporal lobe.

Precautions

The multiple factors that may contribute to brain degeneration over a long period of time need to be carefully considered before a diagnosis of CTE is made.

Management

The development of degenerative processes is more likely with persistent deficits after injury.

These individuals will benefit from periodic reevaluation and care by rehabilitation specialists, and their families will likely benefit from ongoing education, support and, if needed, respite care.

For individuals without significant functional deficits after injury, it is unclear if there are specific rehabilitative interventions to prevent CTE.

Encouraging healthy nutrition with weight management, avoiding tobacco usage, using alcohol in moderation, regular conditioning and functionally-focused exercise, consistent primary medical care, engagement in cognitive stimulating activities, alternating with restorative rest, and maintaining rich social contacts is recommended.

Prevention of repeat injury and other safety issues is also an important aspect of care.

Disability Determination and Medico-Legal Issues

1. Although the vast majority of individuals who sustain polytrauma will have a return to normal or near normal functioning, for those with persistent difficulties, accurate and fair disability determination (DD) is important to optimize their long-term success. Research has demonstrated that many patients are unable to move forward with their rehabilitation activities (especially vocational) until a DD has been made. These patients should be educated on the natural course of recovery after injury, the role of rehabilitation efforts and the DD process. For example, vocational rehabilitation efforts that demonstrate full participation and engagement are more likely to be successful or, if not, to positively

influence a DD. Medico-legal issues related to liability for injury should play no direct role in clinical care or DD; however, they are often quite distracting to patients and their recovery. It is important that DD be determined by a trained professional who is not one of the patient's clinicians (due to ethical and conflict of interest issues) at the point in time when they are reasonably expected to be at maximal medical improvement (MMI; a plateau of improvement that is expected to persist). In general, almost all individuals whose polytrauma injury is predominantly characterized by mild traumatic brain injury (TBI; including postconcussive syndrome), one or more fractures, single limb amputations, or chronic extremity/trunk pain will have reached their MMI by 1 year postinjury. Those with moderate to severe TBI, spinal cord injury, or burns are more likely to need at least 2 years before MMI is reached.

2. An accurate DD relies on the examiner having sufficient knowledge of both the basics of polytrauma injuries and the specifics of the injured individual's issues. The latter may be gleaned by the following:
   - A review of all medical records, including initial injury documentation if available
   - A review of the patient's ongoing symptoms and highest, consistent level of functioning determined by his/her treating clinicians, including vocational specialists
   - A review of the patient's current treatments (DD should be delayed if the patient is still improving with treatment)
   - A review of the patient's home and community functioning from the patient's and caregiver's perspectives

- A detailed examination of the patient, including both a general assessment of health and a specific evaluation of symptoms and functioning
- A review of objective testing of physical, cognitive, behavioral, and functional skills (including those obtained by clinicians and, as needed, by the examiner)

3. The DD should provide an objective description of the patient's physical and functional status, with a clear identification of persistent impairments, symptoms, and disability. Medico-legal issues related to liability for initial or secondary injury should not play a role in the DD; however, it is appropriate for the DD specialist to opine on the relatedness of secondary injury, symptoms, and disability to the initial polytrauma injury. Similarly, the adjudication of benefits (including financial and health care provision) and accommodations (for vocational considerations), which are usually made separately (by a third party) based on the DD depending on eligibility and policy guidelines, should not be influenced by medico-legal issues, unless regulated by eligibility (eg, if the patient's actions or behaviors had a direct role in the initial injury). While the clinical team should provide an accurate representation of the patient's needs and abilities in the medical documentation, taking into consideration the practical application of the patient's deficits and skills, it is not appropriate for the clinician to attempt to directly impact the DD or subsequent adjudication of benefits and accommodations.

Return to Driving

1. Driving is a highly complex and potentially high-risk functional task that requires successful integration of physical, cognitive, and behavioral skills. A return to driving after polytrauma should be overseen by the patient's rehabilitation treatment team and ideally should be managed through a certified driver's rehabilitation program, culminating in an on-road driving test. While driving is not a primary goal after acute polytrauma, it is an integral aspect of successful community reintegration (at least in most parts of the United States) and often a major obstacle to return to vocational and recreational activities.

2. As noted, an assessment of ability to return to driving requires an interdisciplinary approach and should be made under the supervision of a specialty-certified professional. The basic elements that need to be assessed include:
   - Medical status, including presence of seizures, dizziness, pain, and headaches
   - Physical functioning, including vision (scanning, acuity, photophobia), hearing (acuity, tinnitus), extremity and

neck range of motion and pain, motor tone, strength and coordination (including reaction time), sensation, sitting balance, and ability to ingress and egress the vehicle

- Cognitive functioning, including arousal, attention, concentration, memory, and way-finding skills
- Behavioral functioning, including distractibility, irritability, frustration tolerance
- Ability of the patient to operate the vehicle, with or without adaptive devices (eg, steering wheel knob, hand operated brake/accelerator, modified mirrors), at rest and in real world driving settings (including understanding of road signs and signals)
- Ability of the patient to pass a state Department of Motor Vehicle (DMV) driving test (written and road)

3. Driver's training programs focus on the basic elements noted above, incorporating rehabilitation therapies, home- and community-based exercises and activities, repeated driving practice in supervised and controlled settings, and the use of driving simulators for both skills training and assessment (eg, hand-eye and foot-eye reaction and coordination). Unfortunately, driving simulators and driving video games have no direct correlation with the successful ability to return to road driving. All patients who sustain polytrauma and have any significant persistent symptoms, physical impairments, or functional deficits should be formally retested by either a certified driver's rehabilitation professional (who works collaboratively with the DMV) or a DMV instructor.

Return to Driving

Assessment

An assessment of ability to return to driving requires an interdisciplinary approach and should be made under the supervision of a specialty-certified professional.

The basic elements that need to be assessed include:

- Medical status
- Physical functioning
- Cognitive functioning
- Behavioral functioning
- Ability of patient to operate vehicle
- Ability of the patient to pass a state Department of Motor Vehicle (DMV) driving test (written and road)

Precautions

Driving simulators and driving video games have not been proven to predict the success in road driving.

Management

Driver's training programs focus on the basic deficits and driving prerequisites, incorporating rehabilitation therapies, home- and community-based exercises and activities, repeated driving practice in supervised and controlled settings, and the use of driving simulators for both skills training and assessment (eg, hand-eye and foot-eye reaction and coordination).

All patients who sustain polytrauma and have any significant persistent symptoms, physical impairments, or functional deficits should be formally retested by either a certified driver's rehabilitation professional (who works collaboratively with the DMV) or a DMV instructor.

41

Return to Sports

1. Sports participation and exercise are highly complex and potentially high-risk functional tasks that require successful integration of physical, cognitive, and behavioral skills. A return to sports participation and physical activity/exercise after polytrauma should be overseen by the patient's rehabilitation treatment team and should culminate in a series of practice ("scrimmage") sessions with gradual return to formal sports or activity. While a return to sports and exercise is not a primary goal after acute polytrauma, it is an integral aspect of successful community reintegration and often a key desire of the injured individual. While formal guidelines exist for a return to organized athletics at all levels (eg, scholastic, college, professional), unfortunately these guidelines are inconsistently followed and focus on self-report symptoms and basic neurological testing, rarely taking into account the assessment of the integration of the full range of skills required for a safe and successful return. Additionally, these guidelines have been formulated for

individuals with concussion (initial and repeated), but do not address the complexities of polytrauma or the other types of polytrauma injuries. A comprehensive evaluation by a specialty-experienced clinician/team, in addition to following these established guidelines, is always recommended, regardless of the type or degree of injury.

2. Although controlled research is lacking regarding the period of time required between a polytrauma injury and a return to sports or activity, there are widely accepted guidelines that are utilized. For initial concussion without extended (ie, more than 1 minute) loss of consciousness, exercise can commence once symptoms resolve, and a return to full physical activity with total contact may commence after a 1-week period without symptoms and a demonstration of the ability to safely perform all elements of the sport. For initial concussions with a lengthy period of loss of consciousness and for all repeat concussions, exercise can commence once symptoms resolve and a return to full physical activity may commence after 2 weeks of symptom-free demonstration of activity skills; however, noncontact precautions should extend to at least 1 month. For moderate to severe traumatic brain injury (TBI), amputations, burns, and spinal cord injury (SCI), exercise should be encouraged as soon as tolerated after injury and symptoms allow. If there is a desire for a return to competitive or recreational sports activity and the patient can demonstrate the ability to return to full physical activity (which is not usual), then the ability to return to a competitive or total contact level must be individualized, but typically for TBI or SCI, a minimum of 1 year postinjury with normal neuronal and skeletal imaging is the criterion. Patients with amputations and burns, with or without adaptive devices, braces, or prostheses, who

have demonstrated all needed activity and safety skills may return to sports no earlier than 6 months postinjury.

3. As noted, an assessment of the ability to return to sports and exercise requires an interdisciplinary approach and should be made under the supervision of a specialty-certified professional. The basic elements that need to be assessed include:

   • Medical status, including presence of seizures, dizziness, pain, and headaches
   • Physical functioning, including vision (scanning, acuity, photophobia), hearing (acuity, tinnitus), extremity and neck range of motion and pain, motor tone, strength, and coordination (including reaction time), sensation, balance, and the ability to perform the basic and advanced sports- or exercise-specific motions and actions in isolation and in sequence
   • Cognitive functioning, including arousal, attention, concentration, and memory
   • Behavioral functioning, including distractibility, irritability, frustration tolerance
   • Ability of patient to perform the sports- and exercise-specific skills in controlled, simulated game/activity and actual game/activity settings
   • Ability of the patient to pass any sports or exercise activity formal testing required by designated organizations or (aforementioned) guidelines

4. A return to sports and exercise programs focuses on the basic elements noted above, incorporating rehabilitation therapies, home- and community-based exercises and activities, and repeated activity practice in supervised and controlled settings. Unfortunately, sports/exercise simulators and video games have no direct correlation

with the successful ability to return to play or exercise. Patients who demonstrate all the skills needed for a safe return and have had sufficient time for recovery/healing should be encouraged to do so after completion of training. All patients who have significant persistent symptoms, physical impairments, or functional deficits should be encouraged to return to modified sports or exercise activity that they are capable of safely participating in (with adaptive and safety devices, as needed).

Return to Sports

Assessment

An assessment of ability to return to sports and exercise requires an interdisciplinary approach and should be made under the supervision of a specialty-certified professional.

Precautions

Sports/exercise simulators and video games have no direct correlation with the successful ability to return to play or exercise.

Management

For initial concussion without extended loss of consciousness, exercise can commence once symptoms resolve, and a return to full physical activity with total contact may commence after a 1 week period without symptoms and a demonstration of the ability to safely perform all elements of the sport.

For initial concussions with a lengthy period of loss of consciousness and for all repeat concussions, exercise can commence once symptoms resolve and a return to full physical activity may commence after 2 weeks of symptom-free demonstration of activity skills; however, noncontact precautions should extend to at least 1 month.

For moderate to severe TBI, amputations, burns and spinal cord injury, exercise should be encouraged as long as tolerated after injury and symptoms allow. If there is a desire for a return to competitive or recreational sports activity and the patient can demonstrate the ability to return to full physical activity (which is not usual), then the ability to return to a competitive or total contact level must be individualized.

Return to Work

1. Return to work (or other type of productive activity, such as military duty, volunteerism, school) is a key long-term goal for all individuals who sustain polytrauma and should be the focus, along with overall wellness and health, of the rehabilitation team once the acute medical and functional issues have been addressed. Although the vast majority of individuals who sustain polytrauma will have a return to normal or near-normal functioning, a return to work may require specific rehabilitative interventions to be success-fully and durably accomplished. Research has demonstrated that successful return to work is feasible for almost all individuals who sustain polytrauma, including the most severe of traumatic brain injury (TBI) or spinal cord injury, and is best accomplished using the vocational rehabilita-tion (VR) technique known as supported employment (SE). SE is a system of VR that offers support for individuals with disabilities via ongoing employment in integrated settings. SE provides assistance such as job coaches, job development, job retention, transportation, assistive technology, specialized job training, and individually

tailored supervision. Importantly, SE refers to both the development of employment opportunities and ongoing support for those individuals to maintain employment.

2. The rehabilitation team and specialists in SE must have sufficient knowledge of both the basics of polytrauma injuries and the specifics of the injured individual's issues. The latter may be gleaned by the following:
   - A review of all medical records, including initial injury documentation if available
   - A review of the patient's ongoing symptoms and highest, consistent level of functioning determined by his/her treating clinicians, including vocational specialists
   - A review of the patient's current treatments (VR should be delayed if the patient is still improving with treatment)
   - A vocational history of the patient, including specialty skills
   - A review of the patient's home and community functioning from the patient's and caregiver's perspectives
   - A detailed examination of the patient, including both a general assessment of health and a specific evaluation of symptoms and functioning
   - A review of objective testing of physical, cognitive, behavioral, and functional skills (including those obtained by clinicians and, as needed, by the examiner)

3. VR/SE activities should be introduced during the acute rehabilitation phase and then gradually initiated as outpatient/home-based rehabilitation therapies and care are being completed. SE is usually begun well before patients have reached their maximum medical improvement (MMI; a plateau of improvement that is expected to persist), and therefore well before they had a disability determination (DD) completed with associated adjudication of benefits and accommodations. In fact, the outcome of SE is often a key factor in DD and adjudications.

Return to Work

Assessment

The rehabilitation team and specialists in supported employment (SE) must have sufficient knowledge of both the basics of polytrauma injuries and the specifics of the injured individual's issues. The latter may be accomplished by the following:

- A review of all medical records
- Review of the patient's ongoing symptoms and highest, consistent level of functioning
- A review of the patient's current treatments
- A vocational history of the patient
- A review of the patient's home and community functioning
- A detailed examination of the patient, including a general assessment
- A review of objective testing of physical, cognitive, behavioral, and functional skills

Precautions

SE is usually begun well before patients have reached their maximum medical improvement (MMI; a plateau of improvement that is expected to persist), and therefore well before they had a disability determination (DD) completed with associated adjudication of benefits and accommodations.

Management

Research has demonstrated that successful return to work is feasible for almost all individuals who sustain polytrauma, including the most severe of TBI or spinal cord injury, and is best accomplished using the vocational rehabilitation (VR) technique known as SE.

Diagnosis and Management of Common Sequelae of Polytrauma With TBI and Amputation, Burns, or Spinal Cord Injury

Dual Disability—TBI

With SCI, Amputation,

or Burns

1. Polytrauma injuries all involve the presence of a traumatic
   brain injury (TBI) plus at least one other significant
   physical (eg, burn, fracture, soft tissue) injury or psychological (eg, posttraumatic stress disorder [PTSD],
   generalized anxiety disorder) disorder, oftentimes with
   underlying pre-morbid conditions (eg, substance abuse).
   While these multiple factors will typically result in functional limitations that are in excess of either isolated
   injury or even multiple injuries, the brain is usually the
   major affected organ system. In the case of dual disability, concomitant spinal cord injury (SCI), major
   amputation, or partial to full thickness burns provide a
   dramatic increase in overall dysfunction. While research
   is quite limited in the incidence of major dual disabilities,

estimates range as high as concomitant 50% TBI (usually mild) in all SCI and amputations when associated with combat explosion or injury.

2. The rehabilitation of an SCI is highly complex and necessitates a comprehensive specialty team approach with a period of 8 to 12 weeks for the acute, inpatient phase followed by 3 to 12 months of ongoing outpatient and home-based rehabilitation services. While the management of the profound physiologic and physical changes and deficits that arise from any disruption (complete or incomplete) and any level of the spinal cord is challenging for the clinicians, patient, and family, the biggest challenge is the education and training needed to allow for the lifetime of modifications usually required. Both of these components become significantly more difficult with the overlay of the cognitive, behavioral, and physical deficits that accompany TBI. Optimally the specialty SCI team will collaborate with TBI specialty clinicians and teams to develop a consolidated and individualized approach for each patient. Special consideration needs to be taken for the reduced and changing cognitive functioning, the altered ability to regulate behavior, and the deficits of physical abilities that accompany TBI. Oftentimes the SCI rehabilitation process must be extended or staged; therapies and therapy schedules must be modified to allow for variability and limitations in cognitive abilities; behavior management and modification programs must be utilized; and family/patient education and engagement must be intensified and adjusted. Acute and chronic medical and functional complications are more likely with the dual disability of SCI-TBI, and functional independence and a return to productivity is more challenging.

3. The rehabilitation of single or multiple limb amputations after polytrauma is challenging both because of the surgical and psychologic care associated with the loss of a limb(s) and the intensive adaptation and training required to adapt to using one or more prostheses. Oftentimes the specialty amputation clinicians and team overseeing the process will stage care with a relatively brief acute, inpatient phase followed by a staged inpatient or outpatient rehabilitation phase once optimal healing and residual limb preparation has occurred. These challenges and schedules are significantly multiplied when there is a concomitant TBI that complicates all aspects of amputation rehabilitation. The physical difficulties that arise from TBI, ranging from limb weakness and coordination deficits to amplification of pain, will clearly make adaptation to an artificial limb challenging. Oftentimes more difficult are the cognitive (eg, new learning, multistep command following, divided attention) and behavioral (eg, anxiety, stress management) deficits that are common to all levels of TBI severity. As with SCI, optimally the specialty amputation team will collaborate with TBI specialty clinicians and teams to develop a consolidated and individualized approach for each patient. Again, special consideration needs to be taken for the reduced and changing cognitive functioning, the altered ability to regulate behavior, and the deficits of physical abilities that accompany TBI. The amputation rehabilitation process is likely to be extended; therapies and therapy schedules must be modified to allow for variability and limitations in cognitive abilities; behavior management and modification programs must be utilized; and family/patient education and engagement must be intensified and adjusted. Acute and chronic medical and functional complications are more likely with the dual disability of amputation-TBI, and functional independence and a return to productivity are more challenging.

4. The rehabilitation of partial to full thickness burns, particularly when affecting more than 15% of the total body surface area after polytrauma is challenging both because of the surgical and psychologic care associated with burns and the accompanying disfiguring scarring. Oftentimes the specialty burn clinicians and team overseeing the process will stage care with a relatively long acute, inpatient phase followed by a staged inpatient or outpatient rehabilitation period once optimal skin and skin graft healing have occurred. These challenges and schedules are significantly multiplied when there is a concomitant TBI that complicates all aspects of burn rehabilitation. The physical difficulties that arise from TBI, ranging from limb weakness and coordination deficits to amplification of pain, will clearly make the acute and chronic response to burns, skin grafting and scarring more challenging. Oftentimes more difficult are the cognitive (eg, new learning, multistep command following, divided attention) and behavioral (eg, anxiety, stress management) deficits that are common to all levels of TBI severity. As with SCI and amputation, optimally the specialty burn team will collaborate with TBI specialty clinicians and teams to develop a consolidated and individualized approach for each patient. Again, special consideration needs to be taken for the reduced and changing cognitive functioning, the altered ability to regulate behavior, and the deficits of physical abilities that accompany TBI. The burn rehabilitation process is likely to be extended; therapies and therapy schedules must be modified to allow for variability and limitations in cognitive abilities;

behavior management and modification programs must be utilized; and family/patient education and engagement must be intensified and adjusted. Acute and chronic medical and functional complications are more likely with the dual disability of burn-TBI, and functional independence and a return to productivity are more challenging.

Amputation Care and Prosthetic Fitting

1. The rehabilitation of single or multiple limb amputations after polytrauma is challenging both because of the surgical and psychologic care associated with the loss of a limb(s) and because of the intensive training required to adapt to using one or more prostheses. Oftentimes the specialty amputation clinicians and team overseeing the process will stage care with a relatively brief acute, inpatient phase followed by a staged inpatient or outpatient rehabilitation phase once optimal healing and residual limb preparation has occurred. During the acute inpatient phase, clinicians should focus on optimizing the patient's overall health; maximizing the strength, coordination, and use of the unaffected limbs; and preparing the amputated limb(s) for eventual prosthetic fitting and use. Patients must first learn to be as active and independent as possible without a prosthesis, since an amputated limb is rarely appropriate for weight bearing or prosthetic fitting before

6 weeks after injury. Thus, walking/wheelchair propulsion, transfer, activities of daily living (ADL), and other higher-level functional tasks should be the primary focus during acute rehabilitation.

2. Residual limb shaping after amputation focuses on complete wound healing; optimizing skin integrity; applying pressure bandages/elastic shrinkers to reduce edema and begin shaping the limb; gradually exposing the limb to pressure, touch, and other tactile sensations to begin desensitization (and reduce phantom limb sensation); managing pain (including phantom limb pain); strengthening all musculature; and implementing an extensive flexibility and range of motion program for all joints. Phantom limb sensation (ie, feeling that the amputated limb is still present) is normal and typically resolves by 6 weeks postamputation, while phantom limb pain (ie, pain in the removed segment of the amputated limb) is not normal and must be aggressively treated as any other dysesthetic pain. Phantom pain that does not respond to traditional pain management and rehabilitative techniques may be due to the development of a neuroma at the distal residual limb, which must often be injected or incised. Early use of non-weight-bearing sockets and casts is encouraged to both desensitize skin and nerves to the pressure of a socket and to reduce phantom sensation/pain.

3. Patients are ready for progressive weight bearing on preparatory or initial prostheses when there is total skin healing, near total resolution of residual limb edema, and all secondary medical/surgical conditions are stable enough to support the intensive weight bearing and energy requirements of prosthetic usage. These requirements are much diminished in upper extremity amputations, so this

is less of a concern. Prosthetic sockets that allow for total contact are optimal initially to facilitate edema management and to distribute pressures across the largest skin surface possible. At first the prosthesis componentry (eg, joints, terminal devices, mechanisms) should be as simple as possible to facilitate ease of use and to reinforce a positive outcome for the user. Interdisciplinary teams that include physiatrists, physical or occupational therapists (depending on the limb loss involved), a prosthetist, and the patient/family should make these decisions and be open to frequent early adjustments and changes. Successful long-term usage depends on good initial integration between the patient and his/her treatment team and amputation specialists who have an appropriate understanding of the patient's goals, needs, and abilities rather than a fixation with new or high technology.

4. Common challenges that occur with prosthetic fitting include skin irritation/breakdown, musculoskeletal pain and injury with a return to mobility and ADL usage with the prosthesis, intermittent edema and focal residual limb pain (including the development of bony overgrowth at the distal residual limb) with increased prosthesis usage, prosthesis breakage and need of readjustment/repair, and psychological dysfunction associated with loss of limb/ function and the stresses of a return to "normal." These issues are to be expected and can usually be managed by the rehabilitation team, perhaps with the addition of a rehabilitation psychologist. Of note, rehabilitation care must also focus on optimizing the health, strength, and conditioning of the intact limbs and trunk, as these elements must support the amputated limb(s) and prosthetic usage.

Amputation Care and Prosthetic Fitting

Assessment

> Amputation incision must be healed.
>
> Edema should be minimal.
>
> Residual limb should be able to tolerate tapping and pressure.

Precautions

> Initial amputation incision healing requires a minimum of 6 weeks.
>
> Prosthetic wearing must be implemented gradually.
>
> Limb pain usually responds to prosthetic wearing.

Management

> Begin with a total contact socket.
>
> Utilize simple componentry, especially during initial fitting.
>
> Recheck skin integrity after each period of walking or 2 hours of wearing.
>
> In addition to ambulation training, care should focus on optimizing the health, strength, and conditioning of the intact limbs and trunk.

Spinal Cord Injury

1. The rehabilitation of an individual who has sustained a spinal cord injury (SCI) is highly complex and necessitates a comprehensive specialty team approach with a period of 8–12 weeks for the acute, inpatient phase, followed by 3–12 months of ongoing outpatient and home-based rehabilitation services. While successful management of the profound physiologic and physical changes and deficits that arise from any disruption (complete or incomplete) of any level of the spinal cord is an ongoing challenge for the clinicians, patient, and family, another major task is the education and training needed to allow for the lifetime of modifications that are usually needed.

2. SCIs are typically labeled by their specific spinal cord level of injury (cervical level 1–8, thoracic level 1–12, or lumbar level 1–5) and are categorized as resulting in either tetraplegia (cervical spine/spinal cord damage affecting arms and legs) or paraplegia (thoracic or lumbar spine/spinal cord damage affecting the legs) and further

as complete (no feeling or movement of the limbs below the level of injury) or incomplete (some preservation of either feeling or movement below the level of injury). A knowledge of the common medical/rehabilitation issues and the expected functional outcomes of individuals at the different levels and injury completeness are key for clinicians who manage patients with SCI. In general, patients who have an injury affecting cervical level 7 and below can live and mobilize independently, those with an injury affecting thoracic level 10 and below may do some household ambulation with bracing, and those at lumbar level L3 and below can be functional ambulators. Of course, the patient's age, associated medical conditions, and level of completeness will significantly affect these general guidelines.

3. The key medical and rehabilitation issues that must be addressed after SCI are similar to any patient with significant physical limitation after polytrauma, including skin care, neurogenic bladder and bowel, sexuality, abnormalities of muscle tone and strength, decreased and abnormal sensation, musculoskeletal and neuropathic pain, deep venous thrombosis risk, heterotopic ossification risk, and psychological response to injury and disability. Specialized expertise in SCI is required for both the acute and long-term care and management of these issues. Long-term care must include annual reevaluation of medical and functional status.

4. A unique component of SCI care involves the condition known as autonomic dysreflexia (AD), which is a potentially life-threatening condition that occurs most often in spinal cord-injured individuals with spinal lesions above the T6 spinal cord level. Acute AD is a reaction of the autonomic (involuntary) nervous system to overstimulation

characterized by severe paroxysmal hypertension (episodic high blood pressure) associated with throbbing headaches, profuse sweating, nasal stuffiness, flushing of the skin above the level of the lesion, bradycardia, apprehension, and anxiety, which is sometimes accompanied by cognitive impairment. This sympathetic discharge is triggered by afferent stimuli, typically parasympathetic nerve signals from distended viscera (eg, urinary bladder, bowel, gallbladder), noxious stimuli (eg, ingrown toenail, infected pressure ulcer), or nonnoxious skin sensation that originate below the level of the spinal cord lesion and sends messages back to the spinal cord and brain. These signals are misinterpreted and an excess sympathetic discharge results. It is believed that these afferent stimuli trigger and maintain an increase in blood pressure via a sympathetically mediated vasoconstriction in muscle, skin, and splanchnic (gut) vascular beds. Management must be urgent to prevent stroke, myocardial infarction, and death, and includes sitting the patient up (which lowers the elevated blood pressure), relief of the irritant (eg, catheterizing the bladder, relieving tight clothing or skin pressure), and the administration of rapidly acting vasodilators, including sublingual nitrates or oral clonidine. Patients and caregivers must be educated to the signs and symptoms of early AD, as well as therapeutic maneuvers.

46

Burns

1. The rehabilitation of an individual who has suffered polytrauma with burns is highly complex and necessitates a comprehensive specialty team approach with a period of 8 to 12 weeks for the acute, inpatient phase followed by 3 to 24 months of ongoing outpatient and home-based rehabilitation services. The duration, intensity, and types of services needed are largely influenced by the location and severity of burns, the age and general health of the patient at the time of injury, and the comorbid polytrauma conditions. While the management of the profound physiologic and physical changes and deficits that arise from any burn is challenging for the clinicians, patient, and family, the biggest challenge is the education and training necessary to allow for a potential lifetime of modifications that may be needed.

2. Burns are typically categorized by the underlying cause (eg, thermal, chemical, electrical), location, extent, and depth of the tissue injury, along with the secondary burn-related (eg, pulmonary insult) dysfunctions. Burns are

classified as superficial (epidermis), partial thickness (partially to fully eroded dermis layer or serum-filled blisters), or full thickness (fully eroded dermis with subcutaneous fat involvement to full exposure of bone, tendon, or muscle). Location and extent (eg, total body surface area of partial to full thickness) of burns is used to determine mortality risk and to assist in acute fluid and nutritional replacement needs. Meticulous care should be used in assessing and documenting burns to allow for close monitoring of response to treatment and recovery. Weekly photos or pictures with measurements should be recorded.

3. The key medical and rehabilitation issues that must be addressed after burns are similar to any patient with significant physical limitation after polytrauma or major medical/surgical illness, including contracture, effects of immobility, musculoskeletal and neuropathic pain, deep venous thrombosis risk, heterotopic ossification risk, sexuality, and psychological response to injury and disability. Specialized expertise in burns is required for both the acute and long-term care and management of these issues. Rapid and progressive contractures or shortening of the soft tissues (skin, muscle, tendon, ligament) affected by the burns, as well as a result of the generalized and focal immobilization necessitated by the skin grafting, is the major long-term difficulty after significant burns. Soft tissues across a joint are dynamic structures and will remodel in response to activity or lack of activity. In as early as 96 hours of immobility of a neurologically intact and nontraumatized joint, tissues will begin to shorten and present resistance to movement. These tissues will be permanently remodeled after 2 weeks of immobility. In patients who have burns or skin grafts

these changes may occur more quickly. After months of contracted position, nerves and vessels will also shorten.

4. Prevention of immobilization and repeated joint/soft tissue injury, management of inflammation, and optimal functional positioning of joints at risk are the key to avoiding disabling joint and skin contractures. In addition to regular, controlled active and passive movement of all at-risk (ie, immobilized, grafted, burned, traumatized) joints several times daily, clinicians must also focus on appropriate measures to reduce pain that may prevent joint range of motion, managing acute inflammation and injury with local (eg, ice, wrapping) and systemic (eg, NSAIDs) treatments, and ensure that positions of rest are functionally optimized (ie, will allow for functioning if contractures occur) with bracing and other supports. Contracted soft tissue across a joint will improve to some degree (in proportion to the amount of time immobilized) with a gradated and consistent stretching program. This stretching program should include:
   - Meticulous skin care, including regular use of skin lubricants
   - Prestretching application of local (to decrease pain) and deep (to enhance tissue flexibility) heat 5 to 10 minutes prior to stretching
   - Prestretching pain medication (local or systemic) as needed to facilitate compliance
   - Low velocity, long duration stretching to the point of resistance/pain repeated as often throughout the day as feasible
   - Bracing/casting at the newly optimized length (within pain limits) after stretching
   - Repeated daily functional tasks with the affected joint/limb to facilitate stretching and optimize limb usage

5. Surgical "release" of contractures may be necessary if contractures are "hardened" and do not respond sufficiently to a gradated stretching program. This is most commonly needed following full-thickness burns that affect multiple joints and require multiple, often repeated skin grafting with subsequent immobilization. Any surgical intervention must be followed by a comprehensive stretching program.

6. Treatment of the skin of patients with burns and of skin grafting also involves optimization of nutrition and medical health, including the avoidance of tobacco products, local skin/graft breakdown care (regular cleaning, use of antimicrobial dressings, chemical and surgical debridement, use of bio-occlusive dressings), management of local (eg, osteomyelitis) and systemic infection, total pressure relief for affected area, and close monitoring of other at-risk locations. As possible, rehabilitation efforts should be continued to maintain strength and conditioning, to stimulate cognitive recovery, and to optimize behaviors. Importantly, recovery after grafting entails a gradual increase in pressure to the area once the surgical graft has successfully healed. Patients with burns and grafts are at greater risk for recurrent skin breakdown due to the altered skin integrity and associated scar tissue. Once grafts and scars have adequately healed to allow for pressure bandaging and then custom-fitted pressure garments, these should be consistently applied for at least 23 hours daily for a period of up to 18 months to prevent and reduce the hypertrophic (excess) scarring that typically accompanies full-thickness burns.

Burns

Assessment

Determine whether burns are
- superficial
- partial thickness
- full thickness

Determine total body surface area of partial to full thickness burns.

Precautions

Contractures can begin within 2–4 days of injury.

The position of comfort is rarely the position of function.

Management

Meticulous skin care, including regular use of skin lubricants.

Application of local and deep heat 5–10 minutes prior to stretching.

Prestretching pain medication.

Low velocity, long duration stretching to the point of resistance/pain repeated as often throughout the day as feasible.

Bracing/casting at the newly optimized length (after stretching).

Repeated daily functional tasks with the affected joint/limb to facilitate stretching and optimize limb usage.

Deep Venous

Thrombosis

1. Polytrauma injury that results in a prolonged period (ie, more than 48 hours) of partial or total immobilization, results in a long bone fracture, causes significant soft tissue or vascular damage, or causes a moderate/severe traumatic brain injury (TBI) will greatly increase the incidence of a potentially life-threatening deep venous (or vein) thrombosis (DVT). Deep vein thrombosis, or deep venous thrombosis, is the formation of a blood clot in a deep vein, predominantly in the legs. Once a return to regular mobility and activity has been accomplished, the risk of DVT resolves; however, until this has occurred, close surveillance and management are needed. Unfortunately, early DVT does not have consistent or easy-to-recognize signs and symptoms, thus standardized regimens for assessment and prevention must be utilized. History, physical examination, and provocative

testing (eg, Homan's sign) have no role in this process. Nonspecific signs may include pain, swelling, redness, warmness, and engorged superficial veins. A failure to recognize and manage DVT may result acutely in pulmonary embolus (PE) and chronically in postthrombotic (or phlebitic) syndrome. PE is a potentially life-threatening complication that occurs in up to 10% of DVTs and is caused by the detachment (embolization) of a thrombus that travels to the lungs. Postthrombotic syndrome is the result of chronic obstruction of the major veins of a limb, which occurs in up to 1/3 of undermanaged DVT and results in chronic limb edema, pain, and stasis ulcers.

2. While there are a number of DVT clinical prediction rules (eg, Wells score), any individual who has sustained polytrauma that has resulted in a long bone (eg, humerus, femur) fracture, soft tissue requiring major surgical or procedural care, any operative procedure with general anesthesia for greater than 30 minutes, inability to get out of bed or ambulate for more than 48 hours, or a history of DVT should be considered at a significantly elevated risk for acute DVT. Prophylaxis should be begun immediately, unless there is evidence of intracranial or major organ hemorrhage (in which case it should be delayed for 72–96 hours), with either unfractionated, subcutaneous heparin (5000 units every 12 hours) or low molecular weight heparin (LMWH; 30 units/kg every 12 hours) depending on the number of risk factors. Additionally, the prevention options for at-risk individuals include early and frequent active limb movement (as tolerated), resisted calf exercises, graduated compression stockings (to reduce dependent edema), and intermittent pneumatic compression. These interventions should not be performed if a patient is not on heparin prophylaxis and their

DVT status is unknown (ie, they have not been evaluated with duplex Doppler ultrasonography [DDU]). The use of inferior or superior vena cava filters have no efficacy or role in DVT prophylaxis.

3. At-risk individuals who have not been managed with heparin prophylaxis in the first 48 hours after injury should be evaluated with extremity DDU before mobilization of any type. While this is traditionally performed on the lower extremities, one should also consider upper extremity evaluation if there is impaired movement or trauma, as these veins may also be at risk. Individuals who are determined not to have DVT, but continue to be at-risk and cannot tolerate ongoing heparin prophylaxis (ongoing bleeding, heparin-induced thrombocytopenia), should be fully mobilized as tolerated and have serial surveillance every 72 hours with DDU until they are no longer at risk or can tolerate anticoagulation. Regardless of initial injury and risk factors, the overwhelming majority of individuals who sustain polytrauma no longer require DVT prophylaxis past 8 to 12 weeks.

4. Management of DVT or PE is with full dose, subcutaneous LMWH (1 unit/kg in 2 divided doses) for 3 or 6 months. Recurrent DVT requires 6 months of treatment, while recurrent PE is usually treated for 12 or more months. A full return to the rehabilitation mobilization program may begin 12 to 24 hours after the initiation of full-dose therapy. Management of related swelling, low-grade fever, and pain should be symptomatic; however, full activity should be encouraged. Repeat DDU is rarely indicated prior to commencing activity or at the end of LMWH treatment. Treatment should be reevaluated with new onset of swelling, pain, redness, or other abnormality more than 2 weeks after beginning treatment.

5. Postthrombotic syndrome is directly related to the amount of venous obstruction resulting from DVT and is usually the result of no or poor treatment of the acute event (ie, delayed or limited use of LMWH, failure to fully remobilize the limbs). Treatment is focused on relieving acute swelling, with elevation, gradated compression, and close monitoring of skin integrity and pain related to an exacerbation of venous return (eg, long periods of immobility, hanging the extremity down for extended periods, tight-fitting garments or braces). Prophylactic management includes patient education and training, the use of custom-fitted gradated compression stockings, daily visual surveillance of the at risk limb(s) and meticulous skin care.

Deep Venous Thrombosis

Assessment

At-risk individuals who have not been managed with heparin prophylaxis within the first 48 hours after injury should be evaluated with extremity duplex Doppler ultrasonography (DDU) before mobilization of any type.

Individuals who are determined not to have deep venous thrombosis (DVT), but continue to be at risk and cannot tolerate ongoing heparin prophylaxis should be fully mobilized as tolerated and have serial surveillance every 72 hours with DDU until they are no longer at risk or can tolerate anticoagulation.

Precautions

Heparin-induced thrombocytopenia (HIT) is a rare, idiosyncratic reaction to heparin; a complete blood count should be checked within 72 hours of beginning heparin.

Management

Management of DVT or pulmonary embolus (PE) is with full dose, subcutaneous, low molecular weight heparin (LMWH) for 3 or 6 months.

Recurrent DVT requires 6 months of treatment, while recurrent PE is usually treated for 12 or more months.

A full return to the rehabilitation mobilization program may begin 12–24 hours after the initiation of full-dose therapy.

Management of related swelling, low-grade fever, and pain should be symptomatic; however, full activity should be encouraged.

Postthrombotic syndrome is directly related to the amount of venous obstruction resulting from DVT and is usually the result of no or poor treatment of the acute event.

Heterotopic Ossification

1. Heterotopic ossification (HO), often described as the development of osseous tissue in atypical locations (eg, across a joint), occurs commonly following polytrauma, including burns, muscular injury, fracture, amputation, and neurologic injury. While the etiology of HO is unclear, it appears to be an inflammatory response to injury, although the presence, location, and intensity of HO may not correlate with the severity or location of injury. HO presents in approximately 20% of all patients with traumatic brain injury (TBI) or spinal cord injury (SCI) and nearly 1/3 of individuals with burns, amputations, or fracture of the long bones of the lower leg. HO tends to occur in the first 4 weeks after injury, but may arise at any time in the first 6 months postinjury and, once present, may recur for the next 12 to 18 months. HO related to TBI or SCI tends to occur across the shoulder or hips, with burns at the elbows and hips, and in amputations at the end of the residual limb as well as across the hip. Muscular trauma may lead to the development of

boney tissue (an HO variant known as myositis ossificans) at the area of trauma.

2. HO will present with a limitation in active or passive joint motion (related to pain), oftentimes with local swelling and erythema; however, this presentation may be confused with local joint trauma, arthritis, deep venous thrombosis, or early spasticity. The diagnosis of HO is often delayed because plain film x-rays are not helpful for the first 3 to 4 weeks because there is the establishment of the boney matrix without significant calcium deposition during this period. Similarly, early laboratory tests are not very helpful. Alkaline phosphatase will be elevated at some point, but initially may be only slightly elevated, rising later to a high value for a short time. The only definitive diagnostic test in the early acute stage is a triple phase bone scan, which will show HO in the first 1 to 2 weeks of onset. The triple phase bone scan consists of the flow phase (blood perfusion), blood pool (degree of vascularity), and reuptake (bone turnover).

3. Management of HO is unfortunately not well researched and a definitive treatment paradigm is not well defined. While very focal HO (eg, after a total hip replacement or at a distal amputation site) responds well to radiation therapy (one-time dose of 7–8 Gray), this technique has limited applicability to the diffuse difficulties seen in other causes and the potential risks of this technique in younger adults is a concern. Many advocate the use of etidronate sodium (a calcium chelating agent) for 6 to 12 weeks; however, clinicians have found that once the medication is stopped, the remaining matrix rapidly recalcifies. Similarly, early use of anti-inflammatories (NSAIDs) has been recommended; however, the long-term effects may be poor. In all cases, without a

regular program of multiple times daily stretching and positioning of the affected limb(s), the long-term functional results are poor. Unfortunately, this type of range of motion is extremely painful and poorly tolerated by patients, in particular those who have decreased capacity to understand the need for the stretching (ie, those with cognitive impairment) and those with poor frustration tolerance and behavioral control (ie, TBI patients). While premedicating these patients with pain medications, using local therapeutic modalities (eg, heat, ice, massage), and employing pain management strategies may assist in the process, it remains extremely challenging for both the patient and the clinical team. Limitations in joint range of motion are common in patients with extensive HO.

4. Surgical interventions to remove old HO or improve contracted joints from HO is rarely successful and often dangerous, as HO "bone" is always highly vascularized and bleeds tremendously and the HO often reappears postoperatively and further worsens the joint. Adaptive strategies and the use of mobility devices is a better option than surgical intervention.

Heterotopic Ossification

Assessment

The definitive diagnostic test in the early acute stage is a triple phase bone scan, which will show heterotopic ossification (HO) in the first 1–2 weeks of onset.

The triple phase bone scan consists of the flow phase (blood perfusion), blood pool (degree of vascularity), and reuptake (bone turnover).

Precautions

HO's presentation may be confused with local joint trauma, arthritis, deep venous thrombosis, or early spasticity.

The diagnosis of HO is often delayed because plain film x-rays and serum testing results are either nonspecific or show high false-negative rates for the first 3–4 weeks of onset.

Management

Focal HO after a total hip replacement or at a distal amputation site responds well to radiation therapy.

Many clinicians advocate for the use of etidronate sodium (or NSAIDs) for 6–12 weeks; however, others have found that once the medication is stopped, the remaining matrix rapidly recalcifies.

In all cases of HO, without a regular program of multiple times daily stretching and positioning of the affected limb(s), the long-term functional results are poor. Premedicating with pain agents 30 minutes before stretching is vital.

Surgical interventions to remove old HO or improve contracted joints from HO is rarely successful and often accompanied with significant bleeding and post-op recurrence of the HO.

Contractures

1. A contracture is a permanent shortening of soft tissue (muscle, tendon, ligament) across a joint resulting from prolonged periods of disuse and/or abnormalities of muscle tone (hypertonia, spasticity). After polytrauma, contractures are commonly associated with burns, amputations, complex fractures, severe traumatic brain injury (TBI), and spinal cord injury, and create long-term difficulties with a return to physical independence.

2. Soft tissues across a joint are dynamic structures and will remodel in response to activity or lack of activity. In as early as 96 hours of immobility, in a neurologically intact (ie, normal muscle tone and sensation) and nontraumatized joint, tissues will begin to shorten and present resistance to movement. These tissues will be permanently remodeled after 2 weeks of immobility. In patients who have neurologic abnormalities, such as spasticity or altered sensation (eg, Charcot joint), or who have localized joint or soft tissue trauma (ie, burns, fractures), these changes may occur

more quickly. After months of contracted position, nerves and vessels will also shorten.

3. Prevention of immobilization and repeated joint/soft tissue injury, management of inflammation, and optimal, functional positioning of joints at risk are the key to avoiding disabling joint contractures. In addition to regular, controlled active and passive movement of all at-risk (ie, immobilized, spastic, traumatized) joints several times daily, clinicians must also focus on appropriate measures to reduce pain that may prevent joint range of motion, managing acute inflammation and injury with local (eg, ice, wrapping) and systemic (eg, nonsteroidal antiinflammatory drugs [NSAIDs]) treatments, aggressively managing hypertonia and spasticity with local (eg, ice, electrical stimulation, bracing, neurolytic injections), and systemic (eg, antispasmodics) interventions, and ensure that positions of rest are functionally optimized (ie, will allow for functioning if contractures occur) with bracing and other supports.

4. Contracted soft tissue across a joint may improve to some degree (in proportion to the amount of time immobilized) with a gradated and consistent stretching program. This stretching program should include:
   - Meticulous skin care, including regular use of skin lubricants
   - Prestretching application of local (to decrease pain) and deep (to enhance tissue flexibility) heat 5 to 10 minutes prior to stretching
   - Prestretching pain medication (local or systemic) as needed to facilitate compliance
   - Low velocity, long duration stretching to the point of resistance/pain repeated as often throughout the day as feasible

- Bracing/casting at the newly optimized length (within pain limits) after stretching
- Repeated daily functional tasks with the affected joint/ limb to facilitate stretching and optimize limb usage

5. Surgical "release" of contractures may be necessary if contractures are "hardened" and do not respond sufficiently to a gradated stretching program. This is most commonly needed following full-thickness burns that affect multiple joints, ankle joints in patients with severe TBI resulting in a disorder of consciousness and spasticity, and below knee amputations with secondary soft tissue and boney injury that prevents early limb mobilization. Any surgical intervention must be followed by a comprehensive stretching program.

Contractures

Assessment

Soft contractures develop within 96 hours (4 days) of immobility. It may occur earlier in spastic or traumatized joints.

Hard contractures can form as early as 2 weeks after immobilization.

Precautions

Hard contractures can have shortening of neurovascular structures, so stretching must be gradual.

Management

Prevention of immobility and repeated reinjury.

Management of acute inflammation of joint.

Meticulous skin care, including regular use of skin lubricants.

Prestretching application of local and deep heat 5–10 minutes prior to stretching.

Prestretching pain medication.

Low velocity, long duration stretching to the point of resistance/pain repeated as often throughout the day as feasible.

Bracing/casting at the newly optimized length (within pain limits) after stretching.

Repeated daily functional tasks with the affected joint/limb to facilitate stretching and optimize limb usage.

Pressure Ulcers

1. Decubitus or pressure ulcers are localized injuries to the skin and/or underlying tissue usually over a bony prominence, as a result of pressure, or pressure in combination with shear and/or friction. Following polytrauma with prolonged immobility (eg, after severe traumatic brain injury [TBI], spinal cord injury [SCI], or multiple fractures), this will most commonly affect the sacrum, coccyx, heels or the hips, but other sites such as the elbows, knees, ankles, or the back of the cranium can be affected. In addition to presenting significant medical morbidity and putting the patient at risk of systemic infection, decubitus ulcers significantly delay physical activity and functional recovery.

2. The cause of decubitus ulcers is predominantly sufficient pressure (ie, >32 mmHg for >90–120 minutes) applied to soft tissue such that blood flow to the soft tissue is completely or partially obstructed. An added cause often seen in the acute phase of care after polytrauma is shear force caused by patient's being moved or transferred.

These shear forces pull on blood vessels that feed the skin. Other factors that can influence the tolerance of skin for pressure and shear include protein-calorie malnutrition, microclimate (skin wetness caused by sweating or incontinence), diseases that reduce blood flow to the skin (eg, arteriosclerosis), and disorders that reduce the feeling in the skin (eg, SCI, TBI). The healing of pressure ulcers may be affected by the age of the person, medical conditions (eg, arteriosclerosis, diabetes, or infection), tobacco usage, and certain medications (eg, nonsteroidal antiinflammatory drugs [NSAIDs]).

3. Pressure ulcers are classified as superficial (grade I—nonblanching redness over a bony prominence), partial thickness (grade II—partially eroded dermis layer or serum-filled blister), or full thickness (grade III—fully eroded dermis often with subcutaneous fat showing; grade IV—exposed bone, tendon, or muscle). Meticulous care should be used in assessing and documenting ulcers to allow for close monitoring of response to treatment and recovery. Several times weekly photos or pictures with measurements should be recorded.

4. Prevention is the key to the management of the skin following polytrauma. This includes monitoring and supplementing nutritional status aggressively, including regular recording of weights, an assessment of nutritional health via examination and serum analysis, and inclusion of a dietician/nutritionist in the treatment team. While guidelines vary as to the optimum nutritional and caloric needs after different types of polytrauma, in general a high protein, moderately high fat, low sodium diet is appropriate during the initial recovery (ie, 4–12 weeks) period. The skin should be lubricated with a nonallergenic lotion

twice daily and areas of high moisture should receive appropriate care (eg, frequent changing of clothing, talc powder). For patients who are incontinent or have invasive tubes (eg, nasogastric, gastrostomy, tracheostomy), the surrounding skin must be closely monitored and a barrier type lotion/cream applied. The key component of decubitus ulcer prevention is padding of bony prominences and frequent turning (ie, every 2 hours until the patient is able or willing to move spontaneously). As needed, specialty mattresses should be used to reduce baseline pressures; however, these do not obviate the need for turning and meticulous care (and may make other care challenging).

5. Treatment of pressure ulcers involves optimization of nutrition and medical health, including the avoidance of tobacco products, local ulcer care (regular cleaning, use of antimicrobial dressings, chemical and surgical debridement, use of bio-occlusive dressings), management of local (eg, osteomyelitis) and systemic infection, total pressure relief for affected area, and close monitoring of other at-risk locations. As possible, rehabilitation efforts should be continued to maintain strength and conditioning, to stimulate cognitive recovery, and to optimize behaviors. Importantly, total pressure relief must be maintained in the area of ulceration for healing. For non-healing ulcers, surgical "repair" is needed. Recovery after repair entails similar approaches, with a gradual increase in pressure to the area once the surgical graft (usually a myocutaneous flap) has successfully healed. Patients with healed decubitus ulcers or prior surgical flaps are at an even greater risk for recurrent ulcers due to the altered skin integrity and associated scar tissue.

Pressure Ulcers

Assessment

Pressure or decubitus ulcers are classified as:

- Superficial (grade I—nonblanching redness over a bony prominence)
- Partial thickness (grade II—partially eroded dermis layer or serum-filled blister)
- Full thickness (grade III—fully eroded dermis often with subcutaneous fat showing; OR grade IV—exposed bone, tendon, or muscle).

Meticulous care should be used in assessing and documenting ulcers to allow for close monitoring of response to treatment and recovery.

Precautions

The cause of decubitus ulcers is predominantly pressure (ie, >32 mmHg for >90–120 minutes) applied to soft tissue such that blood flow to the soft tissue is completely or partially obstructed.

Management

Treatment of pressure ulcers involves optimization of nutrition and medical health, including the avoidance of tobacco products, local ulcer care (regular cleaning, use of antimicrobial dressings, chemical and surgical debridement, use of bio-occlusive dressings), management of local and systemic infection, total pressure relief for affected area, and close monitoring of other at-risk locations.

Rehabilitation efforts should be continued to maintain strength and conditioning, to stimulate cognitive recovery, and to optimize behaviors.

Total pressure relief must be maintained in the area of ulceration for healing.

IV

Appendices

1. ASSESSMENT OF AGITATION

Agitated Behavior Scale

A 0- to 56-point scale that may be used to measure agitated behavior after brain injury. It may be administered by health care workers at any level of training and family members.

Agitation Assessment	Score[a]
1. Short attention span, easy distractibility, inability to concentrate.	
2. Impulsive, impatient, low tolerance for pain or frustration.	
3. Uncooperative, resistant to care, demanding.	
4. Violent and or threatening violence toward people or property.	
5. Explosive and/or unpredictable anger.	
6. Rocking, rubbing, moaning or other self-stimulating behavior.	
7. Pulling at tubes, restraints, etc.	
8. Wandering from treatment areas.	
9. Restlessness, pacing, excessive movement.	
10. Repetitive behaviors, motor, and/or verbal.	
11. Rapid, loud, or excessive talking.	
12. Sudden changes of mood.	
13. Easily initiated or excessive crying and/or laughter.	
14. Self-abusiveness, physical and/or verbal.	

223 SESSMENT OF AGITATION 223

Agitation Assessment	Score[a]
Total Score No agitation = 14–20; Mild agitation = 21–27; Moderate agitation = 28–34; Severe agitation ≥ 35	

[a] Key:

1 = absent: the behavior is not present.

2 = present to a slight degree: the behavior is present but does not prevent the conduct of other, contextually appropriate behavior. (The individual may redirect spontaneously, or the continuation of the agitated behavior does not disrupt appropriate behavior.)

3 = present to a moderate degree: the individual needs to be redirected from an agitated to an appropriate behavior, but benefits from such cueing.

4 = present to an extreme degree: the individual is not able to engage in appropriate behavior due to the interference of the agitated behavior, even when external cueing or redirection is provided.

2. ASSESSMENT OF AMNESIA, ORIENTATION, ATTENTION, LEVEL OF CONSCIOUSNESS, AND COMA RECOVERY AFTER TBI

Galveston Orientation and Amnesia Test (Developed by Harvey S. Levin, PhD, Vincent M. O'Donnell, MA, and Robert G. Grossman, MD)

Galveston Orientation and Amnesia Test (GOAT) is a 0- to 100-point scale to assess memory and orientation after brain injury, specifically to determine if an individual has recovered from posttraumatic amnesia (PTA). A score of greater than 70 for 3 consecutive days is considered the threshold for emergence from PTA. There is a modified GOAT, with choices, for individuals with expressive aphasia, mutism, or severe dysarthria and for those who are intubated (a score of >60 on 2 consecutive days defines emergence from PTA).

Galveston Orientation and Amnesia Test

Question	Score
1. What is your name? (2 points)	
2. When were you born? (4 points)	
3. Where do you live? (4 points)	
4. Where are you now?	
a. City (5 points)	
b. Hospital (do not need exact name—5 points)	
5. On what date were you admitted to the hospital? (5 points)	

Question	Score
6. How did you get to the hospital? (5 points)	
7. What is the first event you remember after your injury? (5 points)	
8. Can you describe in detail (date, time, companions) the first event you recall after your injury? (5 points)	
9. Can you describe the last event you recall before your injury? (5 points)	
10. Can you describe in detail the last event you recall before your injury? (5 points)	
11. What time is it now? (5 points, remove 1 point for each 30 min incorrect)	
12. What day of the week is it? (5 points, 1 point removed for each wrong day)	
13. What date of the month is it? (5 points, 1 point removed for each date off)	
14. What month is it? (15 points, 5 points removed for each month off)	
15. What year is it? (30 points, 10 points removed for each year off)	
Total score	

Modified GOAT—Provide Three Choices (One Correct) for Each Question

Question	Score

1. When were you born? (4 points)
  a. Correct day/month but 5 years earlier than actual date
  b. Correct date
  c. Correct year but different day/month	

2. Where are you now? (city; 5 points)
  a. Correct city
  b. Local city
  c. Local city	

3. Where are you now? (hospital; 5 points)
  a. School
  b. Hospital
  c. Office	

4. On what date were you admitted to the hospital? (5 points)
  a. Correct date
  b. Correct day/year but 1month earlier
  c. One week prior to admission	

5. How did you get here? (5 points)
  a. Car
  b. Ambulance
  c. Helicopter	

Question	Score

6. What time is it now? (5 points)
   a. Six hours prior to current time
   b. Correct time
   c. Two hours after current time	

7. What day of the week is it?
   (5 points)
   a. Correct day
   b. Two days later
   c. Four days later	

8. What date of the month is it?
   (5 points)
   a. Two days earlier
   b. Correct date
   c. Two days later	

9. What month is it? (5 points)
   a. Four months earlier
   b. Two months earlier
   c. Correct month	

10. What year is it? (5 points)
   a. Two years earlier
   b. Correct year
   c. Two years later	

Total score	

Moss Attention Rating Scale

The 22-item Moss Attention Rating Scale (MARS) is an observational rating scale that measures attention-related behavior in patients with TBI who have emerged from coma (Rancho Los Amigos Scale of IV or greater). Each of the 22 items is rated on 0- to 4-point scale, and the total score is converted to a 0- to 100-point final score. The MARS is useful to monitor progress in therapy and response to specific interventions (eg, medications).

Moss Attention Rating Scale

Please do not leave any items blank. If you are not sure how to answer, just make your best guess.

1 = Definitely false

2 = False, for the most part

3 = Sometimes true, sometimes false

4 = True, for the most part

5 = Definitely true

1. _____ Is restless or fidgety when unoccupied
2. _____ Sustains conversation without interjecting irrelevant or off-topic comments
3. _____ Persists at a task or conversation for several minutes without stopping or "drifting off"
4. _____ Stops performing a task when given something else to do or to think about
5. _____ Misses materials needed for tasks even though they are within sight and reach
6. _____ Performance is best early in the day or after a rest

7. _____ Initiates communication with others

8. _____ Fails to return to a task after an interruption unless prompted to do so

9. _____ Looks toward people approaching

10. _____ Persists with an activity or response after being told to stop

11. _____ Has no difficulty stopping one task or step to begin the next one

12. _____ Attends to nearby conversations rather than the current task or conversation

13. _____ Tends not to initiate tasks that are within his/her capabilities

14. _____ Speed or accuracy deteriorates over several minutes on a task but improves after a break

15. _____ Performance of comparable activities is inconsistent from one day to the next

16. _____ Fails to notice situations affecting current performance, eg, wheelchair hitting against table

17. _____ Perseverates on previous topics of conversation or previous actions

18. _____ Detects errors in his/her own performance

19. _____ Initiates activity (whether appropriate or not) without cueing

20. _____ Reacts to objects being directed toward him/her

21. _____ Performs better on tasks when directions are given slowly

22. _____ Begins to touch or manipulate nearby objects not related to task

Score _____

Orientation Group Monitoring System

The Orientation Group Monitoring System is a reality orientation group for brain injured patients used to improve attention deficits, confusion, and anterograde amnesia during the period of PTA. Seven behavioral objectives are used to define adequate orientation, attention, immediate recall, episodic recall, and the use of memory aids. Daily performance of each of these areas is aggregated to establish a weekly summary score.

Westmead PTA Scale

The Westmead PTA Scale is a set of nine cards with 7 orientation questions and 5 memory items designed to objectively measure the period of PTA. A person is determined to be out of PTA when he/she can achieve a perfect score of 12 on the Westmead PTA for 3 consecutive days.

Glasgow Coma Score

Glasgow Coma Score is a 3- to 15-point score that assesses level of consciousness after a brain injury, examining eye opening (1–4), verbalization (1–5), and motor response (1–6). It is the "gold standard" for acute assessment of injury severity and has been useful as a reliable predictor of initial survival and short-term outcome.

Glasgow Coma Scale

Points	1	2	3	4	5	6
Eyes	Does not open eyes	Opens eyes in response to painful stimuli	Opens eyes in response to voice	Opens eyes spontaneously	N/A	N/A
Verbal	Makes no sounds	Incomprehensible sounds	Utters inappropriate words	Confused, disorientated	Oriented, converses normally	N/A
Motor	Makes no movements	Extension to painful stimuli	Abnormal flexion to painful stimuli	Flexion/withdrawal to painful stimuli	Localizes painful stimuli	Obeys commands

Mild injury = 13–15; Moderate injury = 9–12; Severe injury = 6–8; Very severe injury = 3–5.

Coma/Near Coma Scale

The Coma/Near Coma (CNC) scale was developed to measure small clinical changes in patients with severe brain injuries who function at very low levels characteristic of near-vegetative and vegetative states. Individuals are tested by at least two independent raters and are tested during a period of "awakeness." The CNC has five levels, based on 11 items, rated 0 to 4 that can be scored to indicate severity of sensory, perceptual, and primitive response deficits.

---

1. Auditory
   a. Bell ringing
   b. Command responsivity
2. Visual
   a. Light flashes
   b. Follow face and look at me
3. Threat
   a. Move hand to within 1–3 inches of eyes
4. Olfactory (occlude tracheostomy 3–5 sec)
   a. Ammonia under nose for 2 sec
5. Tactile
   a. Shoulder tap
   b. Nasal swab
6. Pain
   a. Pressure on finder nail
   b. Ear pinch
7. Vocalization (spontaneous)

Level 0 = no coma (score = 0.00–0.89).

Level 1 = near coma (score = 0.90–2.00).

Level 2 = moderate coma (score = 2.01–2.89).

Level 3 = marked Coma (score = 2.90–3.49).
Level 4 = extreme coma (score = 3.5–4.00).

JFK Coma Recovery Scale

The purpose of the JFK Coma Recovery scale is to assist with the differential diagnosis, prognostic assessment, and treatment planning for patients with disorders of consciousness. The scale consists of six subscales addressing auditory, motor, oromotor, communications, and arousal functions, and ranges 0 to 23. The subscales are hierarchically arranged with lowest scores representing reflexive activity and the higher scores representing cognitively mediated activities.

JFK Coma Recovery Scale

Domain	Score
Auditory function scale	
4—Consistent movement to command[a]	
3—Reproducible movement to command[a]	
2—Localization to sound	
1—Auditory startle	
0—None	
Visual function scale	
5—Object recognition[a]	
4—Object localization: reaching[a]	
3—Visual pursuit[a]	
2—Fixation[a]	

(Continued)

Domain	Score
1—Visual startle	
0—None	
Motor function scale	
6—Functional object use[b]	
5—Automatic motor response[a]	
4—Object manipulation[a]	
3—Localization to noxious stimulation[a]	
2—Flexion withdrawal	
1—Abnormal posturing	
0—None/flaccid	
Oromotor/verbal function scale	
3—Intelligible verbalization[a]	
2—Vocalization/oral movement	
1—Oral reflexive movement	
0—None	
Communication scale	
2—Functional: accurate[b]	
1—Nonfunctional: intentional[a]	
0—None	

Domain	Score
Arousal scale	
3—Attention	
2—Eye opening without stimulation	
1—Eye opening with stimulation	
0—Unarousable	
Total score	

[a] Denotes minimal conscious state.

[b] Denotes emergence from minimal conscious state.

3. ASSESSMENT OF BALANCE

Berg Balance Score

A 14-item scale used to assess balance for individuals who are able to stand without an assistive device. Each item is scored 0 to 4, with 0 being the lowest level of functional ability and 4 the highest level of functional ability. It may be used to determine fall risk:

- 41–56 = low fall risk
- 21–40 = medium fall risk
- 0–20 = high fall risk

Berg Balance Score Assessment

Item	Score
1. Sitting to standing	
2. Standing unsupported	
3. Sitting unsupported	
4. Standing to sitting	
5. Transfers	
6. Standing with eyes closed	
7. Standing with feet together	
8. Reaching forward with outstretched arms	
9. Retrieving object from floor	
10. Turning to look behind	
11. Turning 360°	
12. Placing alternative foot on stool	
13. Standing with one foot on stool	
14. Standing on one foot	
Total Score	

Timed Get Up and Go

The Timed Get Up and Go test records the time required to rise from sitting, ambulate a distance (10 ft), and return to the original seated position without the use of an assistive device. It assesses sit to stand, standing balance, gait, and turning balance.

Instructions: The person may wear their usual footwear and can use any assistive device they normally use.

Timed Get Up and Go Test

Note: The person should be given one practice trial and then three actual trials. The times from the three actual trials are averaged.

1. Have the person sit in the chair with their back to the chair and their arms resting on the arm rests.
2. Ask the person to stand up from a standard chair and walk a distance of 10 ft (3 m).
3. Have the person turn around, walk back to the chair, and sit down again.
4. Timing begins when the person starts to rise from the chair and ends when he or she returns to the chair and sits down.
5. Record time in seconds.

Categorizing results:

< 10 sec = freely mobile

< 20 sec = mostly independent

20–29 sec = variable mobility

> 20 sec = impaired mobility

Computerized Posturography

Computerized posturography is a measure of dynamic balance measured during quiet and challenged standing activities measured on a force plate. Posturography may be performed on an isolated force plate with a computerized screen for visual feedback in a testing laboratory/therapy gym or within the confines of a larger assessment unit (eg, Balance Master, Equitest) that allows for variation to the surrounding visual input (eg, background varied to simulate movement).

4. ASSESSMENT OF BOWEL AND BLADDER FUNCTION

Bowel Manometry

Bowel manometry is the measurement of pressures within the lower bowel and electrical activity of the internal and external anal sphincters while varying levels of volume are introduced into the bowel. These values are also measured during defecation. These values are used to assess for causes of constipation and incontinence after traumatic brain injury.

Bladder Urodynamics

Bladder urodynamics is the measurement of pressures within the bladder and electrical activity of the internal and external urinary sphincters during varying levels of volume introduced into the bladder. These values and the rate of flow are also measured during urination. These values are used to assess for causes of urinary retention and incontinence after TBI.

5. ASSESSMENT OF CONCUSSION AND POSTCONCUSSION SYMPTOMS (PCS)

Concussion Grading Scales

Source	Grade 1—mild	Grade 2—moderate	Grade 3—severe	Complicated
American Academy of Neurology	No LOC symptoms < 15 min	No LOC symptoms > 15 min	+LOC	
Colorado Medical Society	No LOC confusion without amnesia	No LOC confusion with amnesia	+LOC	
Aspen Concussion Consensus Conference	No LOC or PTA < 30 min	LOC < 5 min PTA 30 min–24 h	LOC > 5 min PTA > 24 h	
Williams, Levin, and Eisenberg				Evidence of subarachnoid hemorrhage on initial CT scan

LOC = loss of consciousness; PTA = posttraumatic amnesia; CT = computerized tomography.

Suggested Reading

1. Practice parameter: the management of concussion in sports (summary statement). Report of the quality standards subcommittee. *Neurology*. 1997;48:581–585.
2. Colorado Medical Society. Report of the Sports Medicine Committee. Guidelines for the Management of Concussion in Sports. Colorado Medical Society; 1990 (Revised May 1991). Class III.
3. Cantu RC. Guidelines for return to contact sports after a cerebral concussion. *Physician Sports Med*. 1986; 14(10):75–76, 79, 83.
4. Williams D, Levin H, Eisenberg H. Mild head injury classification. *Neurosurgery*. 1990;27:422–428.

Rivermead Postconcussion Symptoms Questionnaire

This questionnaire can be administered to a person who sustains a concussion to measure the severity of 16 different symptoms commonly found after mild traumatic brain injury. The person is asked to rate how severe (0–4) each of the symptoms has been over the past 24 hours compared to how it was before the injury.

For each one, please circle the number closest to your answer
0 = not experienced at all
1 = no more of a problem
2 = a mild problem
3 = a moderate problem
4 = a severe problem

(Continued)

Compared with before the accident, do you now (ie, over the last 24 h) suffer from	
Headaches	0 1 2 3 4
Feelings of dizziness	0 1 2 3 4
Nausea and/or vomiting	0 1 2 3 4
Noise sensitivity, easily upset by loud noise	0 1 2 3 4
Sleep disturbance	0 1 2 3 4
Fatigue, tiring more easily	0 1 2 3 4
Being irritable, easily angered	0 1 2 3 4
Feeling depressed or tearful	0 1 2 3 4
Feeling frustrated or impatient	0 1 2 3 4
Forgetfulness, poor memory	0 1 2 3 4
Poor concentration	0 1 2 3 4
Taking longer to think	0 1 2 3 4
Blurred vision	0 1 2 3 4
Light sensitivity, easily upset by bright light	0 1 2 3 4
Double vision	0 1 2 3 4
Restlessness	0 1 2 3 4
Score _____	

Neurobehavioral Symptom Inventory (NSI)

The neurobehavioral symptom inventory (NSI) is a questionnaire that can be administered to a person who sustains a concussion to measure the severity of 22 different symptoms commonly found after mild traumatic brain injury. The person is asked to rate how severe (0–4) each of the symptoms has been compared to how it was before the injury.

Neurobehavioral Symptom Inventory

For each one, please circle the number closest to your answer

None (0) = rarely if ever present; not a problem at all

Mild (1) = occasionally present, but it does not disrupt activities; I can usually continue what I am doing; does not really concern me.

Moderate (2) = often present, occasionally disrupts my activities; I can usually continue what I am doing with some effort; I am somewhat concerned.

Severe (3) = frequently present and disrupts activities; I can only do things that are fairly simple or take little effort; I feel like I need help.

Very severe (4) = almost always present and I have been unable to perform at work, school, or home due to this problem; I probably cannot function without help.

Compared with before the accident how have you been doing with the following symptoms

Symptom	None	Mild	Moderate	Severe	Very severe
Feeling dizzy	0	1	2	3	4
Loss of balance	0	1	2	3	4
Poor coordination, clumsy	0	1	2	3	4
Headaches	0	1	2	3	4
Nausea	0	1	2	3	4
Vision problems, blurring, trouble seeing	0	1	2	3	4

(Continued)

Neurobehavioral Symptom Inventory (*Continued*)

Symptom	None	Mild	Moderate	Severe	Very severe
Sensitivity to light	0	1	2	3	4
Hearing difficulty	0	1	2	3	4
Sensitivity to noise	0	1	2	3	4
Numbness or tingling on parts of my body	0	1	2	3	4
Change in taste and/or smell	0	1	2	3	4
Loss of appetite or increase appetite	0	1	2	3	4
Poor concentration, cannot pay attention	0	1	2	3	4
Forgetfulness, cannot remember things	0	1	2	3	4
Difficulty making decisions	0	1	2	3	4

Symptom	None	Mild	Moderate	Severe	Very severe
Slowed thinking, difficulty getting organized, cannot finish things	0	1	2	3	4
Fatigue, loss of energy, getting tired easily	0	1	2	3	4
Difficulty falling or staying asleep	0	1	2	3	4
Feeling anxious or tense	0	1	2	3	4
Feeling depressed or sad	0	1	2	3	4
Irritability, easily annoyed	0	1	2	3	4
Poor frustration tolerance, feeling easily overwhelmed by things	0	1	2	3	4
Score					

6. ASSESSMENT OF COGNITION

Rancho Los Amigos Scale, Revised

Rancho Los Amigos Scale, Revised is a 10-level scale that defines levels of cognitive functioning after brain injury. It is used to categorize a person's current status.

RLAS Level of Cognitive Functioning

Level I—no response: total assistance

Level II—generalized response: total assistance

Level III—localized response: total assistance

Level IV—confused/agitated: maximal assistance

Level V—confused, inappropriate nonagitated: maximal assistance

Level VI—confused, appropriate: moderate assistance

Level VII—automatic, appropriate: minimal assistance for daily living skills

Level VIII—purposeful, appropriate: stand-by assistance

Level IX—purposeful, appropriate: stand-by assistance on request

Level X—purposeful, appropriate: modified independent

Neuropsychological Testing

A standardized cognitive and behavioral evaluation using validated and normed testing performed in a formal environment. Testing uses specifically designed tasks to measure a psychological function known to be linked to a particular brain structure or pathway. Neuropsychological tests are typically administered to a single person working with an examiner in a quiet office environment, free from distractions. As such, it can be argued that neuropsychological tests at times offer an estimate of a person's peak level of cognitive performance. While neuropsychological testing can be used to identify types and severity of deficits, there is little relationship between specific deficits identified and anatomic (brain) structures. Typically, individuals who have sustained moderate to severe TBIs have such a wide array of deficits of varying severity that they are unable to fully participate in neuropsychological testing until they have had a period of recovery. As such, only small components of testing may be used to define deficits, and a comprehensive assessment may be delayed until they are being transitioned from an inpatient rehabilitation unit or are looking at resuming some community reintegration (eg, independent living, return to employment). While all neuropsychological testing should be individualized based on the expertise of the neuropsychologist and the specific injuries and needs of the patient being evaluated, a standard, brief (1 h) battery that could be used to assess individuals with persistent mild deficits could include:

- California Verbal Learning Test II—memory measure
- Brief VisuoSpatial Memory Test—memory measure
- Test of Memory Malingering—effort measure
- Wechsler Adult Intelligence Scale IV (WAIS-IV) Working Memory
- Domain score (WAIS-IV): Digit Span, Letter-Number Sequencing, Arithmetic subtests—attention and concentration measure
- Stroop Classic—attention and concentration measure
- Delis-Kaplan Executive Function System: Controlled Oral Word Association (COWA)—language measure

- WAIS-IV Processing Speed Domain score: Symbol Search, Coding, Cancelation subtests—flexibility and processing measure
- Trail Making Test Versions A & B—attention and concentration measure
- Grooved Pegboard—attention and concentration measure

7. ASSESSMENT OF DIZZINESS AND VERTIGO

Caloric Testing

Caloric testing is used to measure the functioning of the labyrinthian system of the inner ear. Pupillary findings (eg, horizontal and vertical nystagmus) and subjective reports of vertigo are recorded in response to cold water injected into the ear canals.

Electronystagmography

Electronystagmography is an electrophysiologic measure of pupillary response to vertical and horizontal visual stimuli.

Dix-Hallpike Maneuver

Dix-Hallpike maneuver is an assessment of the individual's subjective report of vertigo to rapid movement from sitting to lying with head rotated. Used as an assessment for benign paroxysmal positional vertigo.

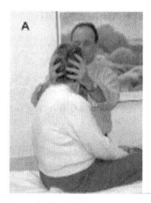 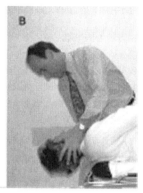

The left Dix-Hallpike test. (A) The patient sits with legs extended on the table and cervical spine rotated 45° to the left. The examiner places his hands on either side of the patient's head, with his right forearm behind the patient's left shoulder. (B) The patient is quickly brought into supine, and the cervical spine extended approximately 10°. The examiner observes the patient for nystagmus and symptoms. With permission from Zasler ND, Katz DI, Zafonte RD. *Brain Injury Medicine: Principles and Practice*. New York, NY: Demos Medical Publishing; 2007.

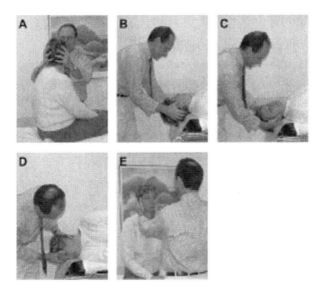

The Canalith Repositioning Maneuver for left-sided benign paroxysmal postural vertigo. (A) The starting position is identical to the initial position in the Dix-Hallpike test, with the cervical spine rotated 45° to the left. (B) The patient is brought into supine, and the cervical spine is extended approximately 10° (45° of left cervical rotation is maintained). (C) The cervical spine is rotated 90° to the right to end up in 45° rotation to the right. (D) The patient is rotated onto the right side, maintaining the cervical rotation to the right. The cervical spine is brought out of extension and is laterally flexed to the right. (E) The patient is brought into sitting. As the patient rises from right-side lying to sitting, the cervical rotation to the right is maintained. With permission from Zasler ND, Katz DI, Zafonte RD. *Brain Injury Medicine: Principles and Practice*. New York, NY: Demos Medical Publishing; 2007.

8. ASSESSMENT OF SLEEP

Multiple Sleep Latency Test

The Multiple Sleep Latency Test is a sleep disorder diagnostic tool used to measure the time it takes from the start of a daytime nap period to the first signs of sleep, called "sleep latency." This test measures "sleepiness."

Minutes to Sleep	Sleepiness
0–5	Severe
5–10	Troublesome
10–15	Manageable
15–20	Excellent

Epworth Sleepiness Scale

This is a patient questionnaire used to measure daytime sleepiness, ranked from 0 (no chance of dozing) to 3 (high chance of dozing), in a variety of settings, sitting and reading, sitting inactive in a public place, sitting as a car passenger for an hour, lying down in the afternoon, sitting and talking to someone, sitting quietly after lunch, and sitting in a car stuck in traffic. It is scored as either "average" (0–9) or "recommend referral to a sleep specialist" (10–24).

Chance of dozing

0 = no chance of dozing

1 = slight chance of dozing

2 = moderate chance of dozing

3 = high chance of dozing

Situation	Chance of dozing
Sitting and reading	
Watching TV	
Sitting inactive in a public place (eg, a theater or a meeting)	
As a passenger in a car for an hour without a break	
Lying down to rest in the afternoon when circumstances permit	
Sitting and talking to someone	
Sitting quietly after a lunch without alcohol	
In a car, while stopped for a few minutes in traffic	
Score _____	

9. ASSESSMENT OF SMELL

University of Pennsylvania Smell Identification Test

The University of Pennsylvania Smell Identification Test is a 40-item smell recognition test via scratch and sniff cards. Normal individuals will score in the 30s (ie, 30 smells detected correctly), individuals with hyposmia in 20s, and individuals with anosmia with scores closer to 10. The cards also include odors that can be detected via both the olfactory and trigeminal nerves to eliminate malingering.

10. ASSESSMENT OF TINNITUS

Tinnitus Handicap Inventory

The Tinnitus Handicap Inventory (THI) is a patient questionnaire consisting of 25 questions answered "yes" (4 points),
"sometimes" (2 points), or "no" (0 points).

1. Because of your tinnitus, is it difficult to concentrate?	Yes / Sometimes / No
2. Does the loudness of your tinnitus make it difficult for you to hear people?	Yes / Sometimes / No
3. Does your tinnitus make you angry?	Yes / Sometimes / No
4. Does your tinnitus make you feel confused	Yes / Sometimes / No
5. Because of your tinnitus, do you feel desperate?	Yes / Sometimes / No
6. Do you complain a great deal about your tinnitus?	Yes / Sometimes / No
7. Because of your tinnitus, do you have trouble falling asleep at night?	Yes / Sometimes / No
8. Do you feel that you cannot escape your tinnitus?	Yes / Sometimes / No
9. Does your tinnitus interfere with your ability to enjoy social activities (such as going out to dinner, to the movies)?	Yes / Sometimes / No

(*Continued*)

10. Because of your tinnitus, do you feel frustrated?	Yes / Sometimes / No
11. Because of your tinnitus, do you feel that you have a terrible disease?	Yes / Sometimes / No
12. Does your tinnitus make it difficult for you to enjoy life?	Yes / Sometimes / No
13. Does your tinnitus interfere with your job or household duties?	Yes / Sometimes / No
14. Because of your tinnitus, do you find that you are often irritable?	Yes / Sometimes / No
15. Because of your tinnitus, is it difficult for you to read?	Yes / Sometimes / No
16. Does your tinnitus make you upset?	Yes / Sometimes / No
17. Do you feel that your tinnitus problem has placed stress on your relationship with members of your family and friends?	Yes / Sometimes / No
18. Do you find it difficult to focus your attention away from your tinnitus and on other things?	Yes / Sometimes / No

19. Do you feel that you have no control over your tinnitus?	Yes / Sometimes / No
20. Because of your tinnitus, do you often feel tired?	Yes / Sometimes / No
21. Because of your tinnitus, do you feel depressed?	Yes / Sometimes / No
22. Does your tinnitus make you feel anxious?	Yes / Sometimes / No
23. Do you feel that you can no longer cope with your tinnitus?	Yes / Sometimes / No
24. Does your tinnitus get worse when you are under stress?	Yes / Sometimes / No
25. Does your tinnitus make you feel insecure?	Yes / Sometimes / No
Score _____	

The THI is graded using the following levels:

- 0–16 = grade 1 (slight)
- 18–36 = grade 2 (mild)
- 38–56 = grade 3 (moderate)
- 58–76 = grade 4 (severe)
- 78–100 = grade 5 (catastrophic)

1. MEDICAL TREATMENT OF AGITATION

Drug:	Haloperidol
Mechanism of Action:	Dopamine antagonist
Dosing:	2 mg initially 10–20 mg daily max dose
Advantages:	Can be given IM or IV. Rapid onset of action ~30 minutes
Disadvantages:	May prolong brain recovery; May cause extrapyramidal symptoms; May lead to akathisia (motor restless-ness); Prolong QT interval; May lower seizure threshold; Neuroleptic malignant syndrome
Drug:	Lorezapam
Mechanism of Action:	GABA agonist
Dosing:	1–2 mg doses
Advantages:	Only benzodiazepine with rapid IM absorption; Few drug–drug interactions
Disadvantages:	Can exacerbate confusion and cause further agitation; May be detrimental to brain injury recovery
Drug:	Olanzepine
Mechanism of Action:	Dopamine and serotonin antagonist
Dosing:	Start 5 mg orally Max oral 10 mg. 10 mg IM for severe agitation. May repeat ×2 every 3 hours
Advantages:	Oral and IM preparations. Rapid onset of action
Disadvantages:	Do not coadminister with benzodiazepines

Drug:	Propanolol
Mechanism of Action:	Beta-blocker
Dosing:	Start 60 mg Max 420 mg
Advantages:	Helps treat symptoms of hyperadrenalism
Disadvantages:	Side effects include sedation, hypotension, and bradycardia
Drug:	Methylphenidate
Mechanism of Action:	Facilitates dopamine and norepinephrine transmission
Dosing:	Start 5 mg twice daily; Average dose 20–30 mg daily; Max 60 mg daily
Advantages:	Helps with concentration
Disadvantages:	Cautions in patients with cardiovascular dysfunction
Drug:	Amantadine
Mechanism of Action:	Facilitates dopamine transmission
Dosing:	Start 50 mg twice daily; Max 400 mg
Advantages:	May enhance recovery
Disadvantages:	May lead to anxiety or visual hallucinations
Drug:	Valproic Acid
Mechanism of Action:	Anticonvulsant
Dosing:	Start 10 mg/kg/d; Max 60 mg/kg/d
Advantages:	Usually effective within 1 week; No significant effect on neuropsychological testing
Disadvantages:	Can cause nausea if not dosed at mealtimes; May lead to pancreatitis or hepatitis

(*Continued*)

Drug:	Carbamezapine
Mechanism of Action:	Anticonvulsant
Dosing:	Start 200 mg twice daily; Max 1200 mg daily
Advantages:	Particularly good effect for irritability and disinhibition
Disadvantages:	May cause motor slowing Can cause aplastic anemia, hyponatremia, and renal failure; Must monitor serum levels; Look out for Stephens-Johnson syndrome
Drug:	Buspirone
Mechanism of Action:	Serotonin agonist
Dosing:	Start 7.5 mg twice daily; Max 60 mg daily
Advantages:	Does not interact with other drugs; Nonsedating; Significant anxiolytic properties
Disadvantages:	May induce seizures
Drug:	Sertraline
Mechanism of Action:	SSRI
Dosing:	Start 50 mg daily; Max 200 mg daily
Advantages:	Helps treat emotional lability
Disadvantages:	2 weeks for clinical effectiveness
Drug:	Citalopram
Mechanism of Action:	SSRI
Dosing:	Start 20 mg daily; Max 60 mg daily
Advantages:	Helps treat emotional lability
Disadvantages:	2 weeks for clinical effectiveness

Drug:	Trazadone
Mechanism of Action:	Serotonin agonist
Dosing:	Start 50–100 mg
Advantages:	Causes sedation and can promote sleep at night
Disadvantages:	May cause serotonin syndrome in patients on SSRIs; Anticholinergic symptoms; Priapism

IM = intramuscularly, IV = intravenously, SSRI = selective serotonin reuptake inhibitor.

Suggested Reading

Lombard LA, Zafonte RD. Agitation after traumatic brain injury: considerations and treatment options. *Am J Phys Med Rehabil*. 2005;84:797–812.

2. MEDICAL TREATMENT OF DEPRESSION

Drug:	Fluoxetine (Prozac)
Mechanism of Action:	SSRI
Dosing:	20–80 mg/d
Advantages:	Low anticholinergic side effects
Disadvantages:	Many drug–drug interactions; Sexual side effects
Drug:	Sertraline (Zoloft)
Mechanism of Action:	SSRI
Dosing:	50–200 mg/d
Advantages:	Low anticholinergic side effects
Disadvantages:	Of the SSRIs, least likely to have a cytochrome-related drug interaction; Sexual side effects
Drug:	Paroxetine (Paxil)
Mechanism of Action:	SSRI
Dosing:	20–50 mg/d
Advantages:	Helps with anxiety
Disadvantages:	Needs to be discontinued slowly; Sexual side effects
Drug:	Citalopram (Celexa)
Mechanism of Action:	SSRI
Dosing:	20–60 mg/d
Advantages:	Few drug interactions
Disadvantages:	Sexual side effects
Drug:	Escitalopram (Lexapro)
Mechanism of Action:	SSRI
Dosing:	10–20 mg/d
Advantages:	Quicker onset of action (1–2 weeks)
Disadvantages:	Sexual side effects

Drug:	Fluvoxamine (Luvox)
Mechanism of Action:	SSRI
Dosing:	50–250 mg/d
Advantages:	Helpful for anxiety and OCD
Disadvantages:	Potentiates theophyllines; Sexual side effects
Drug:	Buproprion (Wellbutrin)
Mechanism of Action:	Inhibits reuptake of serotonin and NE
Dosing:	225–450 mg/d in 3 doses
Advantages:	Less sexual side effects
Disadvantages:	Lowers seizure threshold; Contraindicated in eating disorders
Drug:	Mirtazapine (Remeron)
Mechanism of Action:	Potentiates NE and serotonin
Dosing:	15–45 mg at bedtime
Advantages:	Less sexual side effects; Can promote sleep
Disadvantages:	Very sedating; Weight gain; Risk of agranulocytosis;
Drug:	Venlaxafine (Effexor XR)
Mechanism of Action:	Serotonin and NE reuptake inhibitor
Dosing:	75–225 mg daily if XR
Advantages:	Few drug interactions; Helps with pain
Disadvantages:	Lowers seizure threshold; Increases level of Haldol

(*Continued*)

Drug:	Duloxetine (Cymbalta)
Mechanism of Action:	Inhibits reuptake of serotonin and NE
Dosing:	40–60 mg/d in 1–2 doses
Advantages:	Helps with neuropathic pain and fibromyalgia
Disadvantages:	Contraindicated in uncontrolled narrow angle glaucoma; Caution with hepatic impairment
Drug:	Amitriptyline
Mechanism of Action:	Tricyclic antidepressant
Dosing:	25–300 mg/d
Advantages:	Helps with neuropathic pain; Improved sleep
Disadvantages:	Orthostatic hypotension; Arrhythmias; Can be lethal in overdose
Drug:	Nortriptyline
Mechanism of Action:	Tricyclic antidepressant
Dosing:	25–150 mg/d
Advantages:	Helps with neuropathic pain; Improved sleep
Disadvantages:	Orthostatic hypotension; Arrhythmias; Can be lethal in overdose

NE = norepinephrine, OCD = obsessive-compulsive disorder, SSRI = selective serotonin reuptake inhibitor, XR = extended release.

Suggested Reading

Fann JR, Uomoto JM, Katon WJ. Sertraline in the treatment of major depression following mild traumatic brain injury. *J Neuropschiatr Clin Neurosci.* 2000;12:226–232.

3. MEDICAL TREATMENT OF SPASTICITY

Drug:	Dantrolene sodium (Dantrolene)
Mechanism of Action:	Believed to act directly on the sarcoplasmic reticulum by inhibiting calcium release
Starting Dose:	25 mg orally daily to start; Then increase dose to 2 to 4× per day; May then increase by 25 mg every 7 days
Maximum Dose:	400 mg Doses beyond 200 mg not associated with increases in blood levels, but effect seen
Advantages:	Minimal cognitive side effects
Disadvantages:	Associated with hepatotoxicity
Drug:	Baclofen (Lioresal)
Mechanism of Action:	Active at GABA-B receptor
Starting Dose:	5 mg orally 3 times daily
Maximum Dose:	80 mg daily recommended; Up to 160 mg daily may be considered
Advantages:	Can be given intrathecally for severe refractory spasticity
Disadvantages:	Sedating; Memory dysfunction; May not be as useful for upper extremity spasticity; Abrupt withdrawal can be life threatening
Drug:	Diazepam (Valium)
Mechanism of Action:	GABA-A receptor agonist
Starting Dose:	2 mg
Maximum Dose:	40 mg
Advantages:	Useful for nighttime spasms
Disadvantages:	Sedating; Impaired cognitive processing

(Continued)

Drug:	Clonidine (Catapress)
Mechanism of Action:	$\alpha 2$ receptor agonist
Starting Dose:	0.1 mg daily
Maximum Dose:	0.6 mg
Advantages:	Can help lower blood pressure in hypertensive patient
Disadvantages:	Dizziness; Drowsiness; Hypotension
Drug:	Tizanidine (Zanaflex)
Mechanism of Action:	$\alpha 2$ receptor agonist
Starting Dose:	2–4 mg at bedtime
Maximum Dose:	36 mg daily
Advantages:	Can help with both upper and lower extremity tone
Disadvantages:	Dizziness; Drowsiness; Hypotension Concomitant therapy with ciprofloxacin or fluvoxamine contraindicated
Drug:	Gabapentin (Neurontin)
Mechanism of Action:	Mechanism unknown
Starting Dose:	300 mg orally three times daily; Needs renal adjustment
Maximum Dose:	3,600 mg
Advantages:	Helps ameliorate neuropathic pain
Disadvantages:	Somnolence; Dizziness; Fatigue

Suggested Reading

Davidoff RA. Pharmacology of spasticity. *Neurology.* 1978; 28:46–51.

Index

SETON HALL UNIVERSITY
UNIVERSITY LIBRARIES
SOUTH ORANGE, NJ 07079